FROM THE [...] RUNAWAY BEST SELLERS ARE KNOWN BY MILLIONS FOR THEIR STRAIGHTFORWARD, ENTERTAINING ADVICE

What is the single most important element in your diet?

What is "portion control" in restaurants— and why is it such a rip-off?

Is it true that British fighter pilots outfought the Luftwaffe at night by eating lots of carrots?

What are the amazing similarities between sugar and cocaine?

Why has carrageenin—present in countless "convenience" foods—been placed on the FDA emergency list?

David Reuben, M.D.

Everything You Always Wanted to Know About Nutrition

AVON
PUBLISHERS OF BARD, CAMELOT, DISCUS AND FLARE BOOKS

AVON BOOKS
A division of
The Hearst Corporation
1790 Broadway
New York, New York 10019

Copyright © 1978 by The Maleri Corporation
Published by arrangement with Simon & Schuster
Library of Congress Catalog Card Number: 78-8665
ISBN: 0-380-44370-8

First Avon Printing: September 1979

AVON TRADEMARK REG. U.S. PAT. OFF. AND IN
OTHER COUNTRIES, MARCA REGISTRADA,
HECHO EN U.S.A.

Printed in the U.S.A.

K-R   15   14   13   12   11   10

It should be obvious that nothing in this book is intended as medical advice for sick people. If you are sick, see your doctor right away. But if you want to *keep from getting sick*, eat healthful, unprocessed, uncontaminated food. The publisher also asked me to boldly come right out and say that the medical opinions expressed here are mine and not theirs. That's fine with me. If you look in the front of the book, you will notice that the M.D. comes after my name and not theirs. If the publishers have any medical opinions, they never mentioned them to me.

It's also worth mentioning that *most* physicians agree with the medical opinions expressed here and I would think that *all* of them agree with the medical *facts*.

D.R.

Acknowledgments

I would like to express my appreciation to Don Congdon, my friend and agent, whose guidance becomes more valuable with each book I write.

I would like to thank my good friend, Don José Figueres Ferrer, for all the things he has taught me.

I also wish to thank the Presidents of Costa Rica, Licenciado Daniel Oduber and Licenciado Rodrigo Carazo, for providing the atmosphere of peace and tranquillity that made my work possible.

Doña Marta de Barquero of the Medical Library at the National University provided indispensable assistance in research and source material and helped make this book precise and accurate.

Colonel Guillermo Vargas made life easier in the process of writing, and Licenciado Francisco Morelli proved his friendship many times.

Don Guido Fernandez of *La Nacion* was kind and generous.

Finally, three big kisses for David, Jr., Cathy, and Amy, who gave their Daddy hugs and kisses and smiles whenever he needed them.

*To my wife, Barbara, whose gentle
and loving spirit lives in all my books
—and always in my heart*

Hace mal el que denigra
la Dieta de Alta Fibra
Mal haces tú, cuando de mérito la despojas
yo tengo mi propia receta cabal:
comerse las hojas
y botar el tamal

—JOSÉ FIGUERES FERRER
San José, Costa Rica

Contents

Special Note to Readers

Do you remember the story of the Emperor's New Clothes? Each year, in a far-off kingdom, the Emperor ordered an elegant new wardrobe to parade before his subjects. One year a gang of swindlers took advantage of his trusting nature and sold him clothes that didn't exist —material that was *invisible*. The Emperor was cajoled into agreeing that the nonexistent cloth was beautiful, expensive, and elegant. He paid an exorbitant price for his "new clothes," pretended to put them on, and paraded before his subjects *stark naked*. Everyone was too ashamed— or too proud—to admit that the too-trusting Emperor had been swindled by a bunch of tricksters. As a result they all told him how wonderful his "new clothes" were. Everyone, that is, except for one little boy who observed the Emperor incredulously and finally said: "Your Majesty, you're naked!"

This book was written by that little boy. You have been tricked into liking a breakfast of artificial-imitation-synthetic orange drink, imitation white bread, imitation butter (margarine), imitation jam (made with corn syrup), chemicalized coffee with imitation cream, and possibly imitation eggs and imitation bacon—two "new" products. You gulp artificial-imitation-synthetic vitamin and mineral pills covered with saccharin and artificial colors. You eat 5000 different synthetic chemicals in your day-to-day diet, and you consume more than six pounds of exotic preservatives and artificial chemical compounds every year. You suffer from an epidemic of obesity, heart attacks, diabetes, and cancer unheard of in the history of the world—most of which comes from your rotten diet. The gigantic food processors and food sellers spend more than two billion dollars a year to tell you how well you are eating and how nutritious your awful artificial-chemical-laden diet is.

In this book I am going to tell you in detail—supported by the latest scientific evidence—that you have been sold the Emperor's new clothes. Penny for penny and pound for pound, you eat one of the worst diets in the world—and it is hurting you and your children more than you are willing to admit.

Before you say yes or no, slide your hands down over your stomach and see how much fat you carry there. Run your tongue over your teeth and check the number of cavities—and plastic imitation teeth—your overrefined diet has brought you. Think of your friends and relatives with cancer, diabetes, and heart attacks—and think of the rotten food they ate to get that way.

Then realize that many people on this planet eat better than you do, pay less for their food, have good teeth, slim bodies, and much less diabetes, cancer, and heart attacks. They know something that you don't know: your body —and your mind—is only as good and as wholesome as the food you put into it. The food processors spend their billions to tell you that your body doesn't know the difference between a real strawberry and ethyl-3-methyl-3-phenylglycidate, a common imitation strawberry flavoring. Your body *knows* the difference. And someday when you suddenly wake up with a lump you never had before or a pain that won't go away from the 5000 synthetic chemicals in your food, write a letter to the big food companies or to the FDA and ask them to take care of your family. Good luck.

It is incomprehensible to me that intelligent people have not made the obvious, glaring "Emperor's-new-clothes" connection between the chemicalized, denutrified, contaminated, deeply embalmed garbage we incorrectly refer to as a "modern diet" and the directly resulting diseases that *each year kill more than twice as many Americans as perished in all the many wars the United States has ever fought.* People of America—the greatest threat to the survival of you and your children is not some terrible nuclear weapon. *It is what you are going to eat from your dinner plate tonight.*

That's what this book is all about.

An Open Letter to My Fellow Physicians

December 15, 1977

Dear Colleagues:

First of all I want to thank you for the unprecedented support and encouragement you have given my recent book, *The Save-Your-Life Diet*. I appreciate the thousands of letters, telephone calls, and personal visits. Nothing is more gratifying to me than to know I have been able to help you to help your patients and their families—except perhaps the knowledge that I have helped you and your families—to better health.

I have always felt—and I know you feel the same—that we have a very special responsibility to stand between our patients and the sellers of products. No matter how responsible a drug company may be, we must evaluate the safety and usefulness of every drug in relation to the health of the patient. On the whole there is no doubt that we have done an excellent job.

But there is a whole category of substances that have a far more intense effect on our patients than drugs. That category is *food*—and through no fault of our own, we have neglected that particular area of medicine. Our medical education neglected it, our internships neglected it, and our residencies neglected it. And for good reason—we had to take care of great masses of sick people.

But now it is becoming obvious, with each successive

issue of our most responsible medical journals, that many of these "sick people" are sick specifically because of what they are eating—or not eating. It is also becoming glaringly obvious that each of your patients ingests a wider variety of organic chemicals in one day in his daily diet than he gets by prescription in a year. Furthermore we know that the doses are far from homeopathic, especially when it comes to certain preservatives, coloring agents, and sweeteners.

In my personal opinion, we as physicians are far more qualified to advise our patients on diet than the food processors, newspaper food editors, so-called nutritionists, and even hospital dietitians. But unless we take the initiative, our patients will seek the advice of those who are less qualified. (Grotesquely, one of the few criticisms of *The Save-Your-Life Diet* was that I was unqualified to give dietary advice since I was not a "graduate dietitian.")

Please don't be afraid to tell your patients not to eat so-called enriched white bread. Please don't be afraid to tell them that refined sugar in doses of 150 pounds a year will harm them seriously. Please don't be afraid to tell them that refined flour will damage them permanently. Please don't be afraid to tell them that the money they spend on vitamin and mineral supplements is, for the most part, wasted.

Why should you get involved? Because food processors and sellers are spending over two billion dollars each year in advertising to usurp your role as the principal health adviser to your patients. You have seen the ads that tell your patients first to swallow a nostrum iron tonic—and then when their leukemia exacerbates, consult their family physician. Have you seen the margarine ads that imply you want your patients to eat that brand of margarine? Have you seen the vitamin pill ads that imply that you advise all your patients to pop vitamins every day? Have you seen the imitation egg advertising that hints broadly that if you don't tell your patients to eat the stuff you are guilty of malpractice?

I know that I resent being manipulated that way, and I think you do too. So I invite you to take the leading role in advising your patients how to avoid illness and disability by providing their body with only wholesome uncontaminated food. I thank you for helping them—and they will too.

When your patients bring you this book to read, as they will, please consider carefully the relationship between refined sugar and diabetes, between chemicals in the diet and cancer, and between high salt intake and high blood pressure. In simply these three areas we can save so much suffering and personal loss with such a small exertion of effort.

If you have any questions or if you wish to discuss any specific points with me, I would be delighted to have you write me at the following address:

Dr. David Reuben
c/o Don Congdon
Harold Matson Co., Inc.
22 East 40th Street
New York, N.Y. 10016

Thank you for taking the time to read this letter.

Fraternally yours,

David Reuben, M.D.

DRR/bnh

CHAPTER I
Vitamins—Part One

What are vitamins?

Vitamins are everything—and nothing. Once all the high-pressure advertising and farfetched claims are stripped away, vitamins emerge as what they really are: everyday chemicals found in minuscule amounts in almost everything you eat. Vitamins are so common that it is almost impossible to get them *out* of food. (The closest anyone has come so far to "vitamin-free" dishes is white flour, white rice, white cornmeal, white sugar, and all the other overprocessed food.)

Even more important, if you heaped up all the vitamins you need each day in a pile, that pile would be smaller than the period at the end of this sentence. To look at it another way, divide an ounce into 1000 parts: your maximum vitamin requirement is a mere 7 of those parts every 24 hours. You could store all the vitamins you need each year in a thimble—and still have plenty of room left over.

If the amount is that small, maybe a person doesn't really need vitamins?

No, everybody really needs vitamins. They play an indispensable role in millions of everyday chemical reactions that occur in the body. Every important event, from digestion to reproduction to reading to walking, requires one vitamin or another. If you were to eat a diet *totally* lacking in vitamins, your life expectancy would be measured in weeks, if not days.

Who discovered vitamins?

That's like asking, "Who discovered sex?" Nobody *discovered* vitamins—they were always there. People have been taking vitamins—and benefiting from them—for as long as they have been eating food. (Actually you can't eat any *natural* food without getting a massive dose of vitamins.) The chemists who get the credit for discovering vitamins—especially in old movies on television— didn't discover them at all. What they *did* discover is two things that a lot of people who had never even been to college knew all along:

1. If some important food element is taken out of your diet, you get sick.
2. If that missing element is put back in again, you get well.

That's really all there is to the whole vitamin business —and selling vitamins is one of the country's biggest *and least essential* businesses.

Why do you say that selling vitamins is nonessential?

Just think about it a minute. For over 50,000 years the human race has flourished—long before there was ever such a thing as a vitamin pill and long before the word *vitamin* ever existed. Even today, man's nearest relatives —monkeys, apes, and the rest of the simians—thrive without gulping pills of any kind—and they are healthier than most Americans! The reason is obvious: God, in His infinite wisdom, has provided everything that His children need, including vitamins in their daily diet. The only way a normal person can develop a vitamin deficiency is to deliberately consume only food that has important vitamins removed from it.

And the vitamin scientists didn't do so well either. The history of vitamin research reads like it was written by a mental defective on a slow day. It is a chronicle of stupidity and ignorance—unequaled in the annals of science.

That's a pretty strong accusation. Is there any proof?

There's plenty of proof. Take this example: When the Dutch took the island of Java away from its inhabitants in the seventeenth century, they soon encountered an epidemic of a fatal disease called *beriberi*. This condition attacks the brain and nervous system, the heart and the digestive system. Literally thousands of men, women, and children died each year from the Javanese epidemic. Dutch doctors were helpless; all they managed to do was observe that the condition only attacked the Dutch and Javanese who followed the Dutch customs—including several thousand Javanese who were locked up in a new Dutch prison.

Every Dutch doctor seemed to have his own theory. Some insisted beriberi was a fungal disease; others blamed it on the "damp air," and a few even attributed it to eating fish! The smartest of the group popped up a long time later, a young scientist named Christiaan Eijkman, and he was just as wrong as the older doctors. He thought the disease was caused by a new little animal called a "germ" which had recently been discovered. So Christiaan wasted years injecting blood from beriberi victims into chickens, trying to infect them. The fact that none of the chickens got beriberi apparently didn't bother him—he just kept plugging along. One fateful morning Dr. Eijkman woke up and found that all his chickens were staggering around the yard like feathered drunks. Every one of them had come down with beriberi—even the ones who hadn't been injected with the blood from people who had the disease.

And that's how Dr. Eijkman discovered a cure for beriberi?

Not exactly. That's how Dr. Eijkman's houseboy discovered a cure for beriberi—or more precisely, discovered a non-cure for a non-disease. You see, Dr. Eijkman had been so wrapped up in his wrongheaded research that he'd neglected to give his houseboy money to buy chicken feed. The poor boy had been keeping the chickens going on *leftovers from the good doctor's dinner table; that's why they got sick.* The difference between chicken feed and the elegant cuisine of a Dutch colonist was the difference between life and death.

What was in the chicken feed that was so important?

Actually it was *what wasn't in the white rice* that was vital. The Dutch fed their chickens on grain that wasn't fit, as far as they were concerned, for human consumption. They gave the hens and roosters unpolished or brown rice —the same low prestige food that the natives ate. The Dutch—and the Javanese who ate like their conquerors— consumed fluffy white rice. The houseboy proved to the Dutch doctor what millions of "natives" had known for thousands of years: if you eat white rice instead of brown rice you get very sick. In modern medical terms, which don't say it any better, it goes like this: "Beriberi is a vitamin deficiency which affects only populations subsisting on white rice."

Once the Dutch discovered that white rice caused beriberi, they switched to brown rice?

Oh, no. Eijkman published his work (or rather the work of his houseboy under the Eijkman name) in 1890, and for the next twenty years it was roundly ridiculed. He was relentlessly attacked by the Dutch medical "experts" who insisted that something as beautiful and fluffy as white rice couldn't possibly cause an ugly disease. They continued to concentrate on such "obvious" causes as swamp gas and other "scientific" explanations.

But all was not lost. About 1911, Casimir Funk, a Polish chemist trained in Germany and working in England, read about Eijkman's observations. Dr. Funk may not have been an original thinker, but he knew a good thing when he saw it. He spent the next four months refining almost a ton of rice. He took the polishings off each rice grain and concentrated them until he had a mere six ounces of an almost pure chemical. The rest is history.

Dr. Funk made a new discovery?

No. He got into a new business. He recovered the discarded vitamin from refined rice and named it *vitamine*. The name came from two words: *vita* meaning "life," and *amine* referring to a category of chemical substances composed of nitrogen and hydrogen. Funk was wrong about the name—most vitamins are not amines. Dr. Funk was *not* wrong about the gullibility of Americans. He moved to the United States, started a big vitamin business and became very rich. He established the basic principle of the vitamin business: *"Sell at a high price, with inflated claims, something that everyone can get free."*

Isn't that unfair?

Judge for yourself. Funk's famous *vitamine* (now shortened to *vitamin*), in reality *thiamine,* is available at no extra cost in every piece of meat, every grain of brown rice, whole wheat products, oatmeal, bran, *and almost every other food.* Thiamine deficiencies are unknown in normal people because you can't get the vitamin (also known as vitamin B_1) out of your food unless you do something crazy to it—like refining away the good parts and eating the bad parts.

Who would do that?

The food processors of America do it every day. They take a grain of wheat and at great expense disassemble it. With giant machines that consume massive amounts of costly energy, they separate the wheat germ and the bran from the starchy inner part called the *endosperm*. The bran and wheat germ are just loaded with thiamine, plus many other vitamins and minerals. They are fed to chickens and hogs. The endosperm, which is relatively worthless, is made into white bread, pastry, and spaghetti for you and your kids. These commercial products are so devoid of any food value that your government—*under threat of imprisonment*—forces millers to put back some of the vital substances they took out. Specifically about twenty-four naturally occurring nutritional elements are removed in processing food grains. About six inferior synthetic nutrients are tossed into the product as an afterthought. And remember that you pay both ways: to have the good part taken out and the artificial vitamins put back in. But don't complain too much, because if you didn't pay to have that overprocessed flour "enriched," you and your children just might end up with beriberi.

But isn't it important to take thiamine in tablets?

It's important to the companies that sell the tablets. A tablet containing two milligrams of thiamine hydrochloride (vitamin B_1) sells for about two cents. That means your B_1 tablets cost you a mere $4600 a pound. Considering that the wholesale price of thiamine is well under $10 a pound, there is a nice profit in selling these little pills. Even one halfway decent meal a day gives you—free of extra cost—more B_1 than you need. Judge for yourself the importance of popping thiamine tablets—or any other vitamins for that matter.

What about all the research that proves you need vitamins?

What about it? For one thing, almost all vitamin research is done upside-down and backward. Say, for example, a researcher wants to know the effects of vitamin A. He puts a group of little mice in cages and feeds them a totally unnatural diet that is deliberately deficient in that vitamin. Then he waits until the mice get sick, and carefully writes down a description of their symptoms. Some of the mice might get dryness of their little mouse-skins. The experimenter dutifully reports: "Lack of vitamin A causes dry skin!" That immediately puts him in the same category as his fellow researcher who studied the reactions of a smaller animal, the flea.

How come?

Many years ago, one of the pioneers in flea research performed what is still the classical experiment in that area. Determined to know the effect of cutting off each of the flea's eight legs in succession, he set about the task. Using a flea which he had painstakingly trained to leap into the air on command, he cut off the first leg. He then shouted, "Jump!" As each leg was severed, the flea obeyed as best he could until finally the last leg was cut off. In spite of repeated instructions, the flea did not jump. The researcher carefully noted in his case book: "Cutting off all a flea's legs makes him deaf!"

It *is* true that lack of vitamin A causes dry skin in tiny mice. It is also true—perhaps only by coincidence—that lack of vitamin A causes dry skin in humans. But there are also over twenty-six other causes of dry skin in men and women, including things that never affect mice, like laundry detergents, food allergies, drugs, and even *too much* vitamin A! None of this gets into the vitamin pill ads which announce: "Vitamin A helps prevent dry skin!" The missing half of that statement is: ". . . only if you happen to have dry skin caused by deficiency of vitamin A!"

7

Those kinds of vitamin studies are important only to those consumers who have gray fur, a long tail, live in a cage, have a chemical company for a cook and a Ph.D. for a waiter. They are totally unnatural experiments designed to demonstrate all the bad things that happen if you are *deprived* of vitamins. It is not scientifically accurate to reason upside-down and backward and conclude that if you *consume* vitamins (instead of avoiding them), all the bad things that happen to mice will be replaced by the good things that will happen to you.

There's one other fact that brings the picture clearly into focus.

What's that?

The fact that *no mouse in the world ever suffers from a vitamin deficiency*—unless he is fed specially overrefined food from which the vitamins have been deliberately removed. And that's exactly the same way that human beings get vitamin deficiencies.

The truth is that vitamin deficiency diseases are so rare in the United States that most doctors have never seen a case in their entire professional careers! And it isn't because Americans pop vitamin pills to the tune of millions of dollars a year. It's because you can't get away from those little chemicals called vitamins.

Let's go back to the example of vitamin A. You can get your daily dose of vitamin A from a vitamin A pill that costs about five cents, contains 10,000 units of the vitamin (and nothing else), and is supposed to supply about twice the daily requirement. Or you can eat 1 ounce of fried liver, costing about five cents. That supplies 15,000 units of vitamin A *in the fresh natural state,* plus 7.5 grams of protein, 3 milligrams (mg) of calcium, 136 mg of phosphorus, 2.5 mg of iron, 108 mg of potassium, almost 100 micrograms of thiamine, 1.2 mg of riboflavin, nearly 5 mg of niacin, and about 8 mg of vitamin C! You could also get your vitamin A from 3 ounces of beet greens and get most of the other nutrients at no extra cost.

That's the point: *every vitamin, every mineral, every*

substance required for perfect health can be obtained from the food you eat if you can get hold of food before the processors get hold of it. If you reflect on it for a moment, it has to be that way. Men and women have been getting all the vitamins and minerals they needed long before the first bottle of vitamin pills ever crossed the drugstore counter. None of the advanced (or for that matter primitive) ancient cultures of the world have recorded significant cases of vitamin deficiencies. That includes the ancient Chinese, ancient Hebrews, ancient Greeks and Romans, Inca, Maya, and Aztec cultures, and even the American Indians. The only episodes of vitamin deficiencies in ancient times were exactly the same situations that occur nowadays: wars, famine, and natural disasters. No person consuming a natural unprocessed diet need fear a vitamin deficiency.

There are over two billion people in this world who will never even *see* a vitamin pill, yet they will live long and healthy lives. Ironically at least *half a billion* of them will have greater life expectancies than vitamin-gulping Americans, and without the so-called magic of modern medicine.

But isn't it true that government studies have proved that "millions of Americans have vitamin deficiencies"?

That's what the studies said—but what they didn't say, understandably, was that these "millions of Americans" are in less danger from these so-called deficiencies than they are from, say, dandruff or tight shoes. This is the way it works. In 1972 the U.S. Department of Health, Education and Welfare published a five-volume treatise called *Ten-State National Nutrition Survey,* which purported to show that millions of Americans were deficient in vitamin A. But there was something funny going on. Millions of Americans were not staggering into doctors' offices twisting with the agonies of vitamin A deficiency. Were they ashamed because they hadn't been popping their vitamin pills? Or were they all consulting Christian Science practitioners instead of medical doctors? *Or could it be that these "millions of vitamin-deficient Americans" didn't exist?* The truth is: they *existed* and they *didn't exist.*

How could that be?

A simple—and not accidental—twist of words. The words involved are *clinical* and *laboratory.* If a researcher in some university takes a blood sample from a person and finds that the individual has less vitamin A in his blood than some textbook says he should, that individual is considered to have a *laboratory deficiency of vitamin A,* even though he has no signs of illness whatsoever. In those cases the only real deficiency that exists is a deficiency of common sense on the part of the vitamin researchers. The truth is that nobody really understands what goes on with those obscure chemicals known as vitamins. On the other hand, if a person has a skin irritation, inflammation of the eyes, and visual defects *plus* low levels of vitamin A in the blood that suggests—but does not prove—that he suffers from a *clinical* (or *actual*) vitamin A deficiency. It was this confusion of findings that made the National Nutrition Survey a total fiasco, culminating in the angry resignation of its director. But the damage was done.

What damage?

The vitamin vendors began quoting "an official U.S. government study" to prove that the nation was being ravaged by vitamin deficiencies. (What else?) But that's not true.

The truth is that less than 0.1 percent of Americans are truly deficient in vitamins—and no bottle of Super-Atomic-Vitamins-With-Multiminerals from the supermarket is going to help them. These unfortunates include alcoholics, drug addicts, and patients with severe digestive illnesses that interfere with absorption of their food. For the other 99.9 percent of Americans, most of the dollars *they* spend on vitamins go right down the toilet.

Down the toilet?

That's where it goes. The majority of vitamins consumed —including *all* the B vitamins and every bit of vitamin C— are the kind that dissolve in water. That means that once your body takes out its tiny daily requirement of these very expensive chemicals, all the rest goes bubbling out in your urine. On any given day there are more vitamins in the sewers and septic tanks of America than in the drugstores.

Of course, there are a few vitamins that can't be dissolved in water.

What happens to those?

They are stored in the body fat for use later on. They include vitamins like vitamin A, vitamin D, vitamin E, and vitamin K. These are probably the most promoted, most exploited, most profitable, and least understood of all vitamin substances. Like all the rest of the vitamins, they are merchandised under the banner of fear and ignorance. Either you take A, D, E, and K pills or you endanger "your eyes, your bones, your heart (and organs more vital), and your life-giving blood."

Let's start in alphabetical order with vitamin A. As usual it begins with a myth.

What's the myth?

Back in 1940 when the German Luftwaffe was destroying London by relentless and methodical bombing, the Royal Air Force suddenly got the upper hand, particularly in night air battles. The rigidly censored British newspapers gleefully revealed to all the world that the British advantage was the result of feeding carrots—supposedly rich in vitamin A—to the fighter pilots to prevent "night blindness." From that moment on, a generation of American youngsters were conscientiously overdosed with raw carrots to protect them from night blindness, a disease that has not been a serious threat since the year 1349, when an epidemic occurred in Holland. Even more important, the newspaper reports were all lies—the British had a new discovery called *radar* and were destroying the German bombers electronically, something all the carrots in the world couldn't accomplish. (As a matter of fact, carrots do not contain even the tiniest speck of vitamin A—but more about that later on.)

In any event, like every other vitamin deficiency, you have to really work at it to develop a deficiency of vitamin A. Actually there are three ways to keep from getting enough of that vitamin.

What are they?

Eat nothing but cereal for six months, spend a couple of years in a concentration camp, or suffer from some very serious diseases including cirrhosis of the liver, ulcerative colitis, and other conditions. (Under those circumstances, lack of vitamin A would be the least of your problems.) In reality you could go for at least three months without consuming any vitamin A whatsoever, since a quarter year's supply is already stored in the liver. But that's beside the point—any remotely rational diet has enough vitamin A for ten people. Taking the recommendation of the National Academy of Sciences–National Research Council (USA), which tends to be very generous, the average adult needs 5000 international units of vitamin A a day. For vitamin A, an international unit is about three tenths of one millionth of one thirtieth of an ounce. So the yearly requirement of vitamin A for a thousand people weighs in at barely one pound. You may have had your vitamin A today without even knowing it.

What foods contain vitamin A?

A lot of them. One stalk of broccoli, one-third cup of spinach, half a sweet potato, or one-third ounce of beef liver will load you up with more vitamin A than you can use. Taking into consideration that you can store the chemical in your liver for three months—at least—a couple of ounces of fried liver a week will be more than enough. Vitamin A does not dissolve in water, so the excess is stored instead of being urinated away. However, carrots contain no vitamin A at all.

But all the books say that you should eat carrots for vitamin A—are they wrong?

Yes and no. Vitamin A exists in two forms—*retinol,* from animal tissue, and *carotene,* from plant sources. Retinol is vitamin A; carotene is really *pre*vitamin A and must be converted to actual vitamin A in the small intestine. That process takes about six to eight hours. So carrots contain only the building blocks of vitamin A— your body does the rest. That's good to know when it comes to vitamin A poisoning.

Can you get poisoned from vitamin A?

Well, that's what the Food and Drug Administration thinks anyway. *Theoretically* someone who takes 100,000 international units of the vitamin daily for six months or so can get sick. But not 20 cases a year are reported among 220 million people, and hardly anyone has ever been known to die from too much vitamin A. The most dramatic cases are those of starving Arctic explorers, who in desperation sometimes kill seals and polar bears and eat the animals' livers. They get a dose of about five million units of vitamin A all at once. Within a few hours they get a headache, nausea, and sometimes even throw up. In a couple of days they usually feel better, although they generally lose their taste for any kind of liver.

The FDA, in its infinite wisdom, makes it a criminal offense to sell tablets that contain over 10,000 units of vitamin A—to prevent overdoses. However, a pound of beef liver contains over 250,000 units and a pint of cod liver oil has over a million units. So the opportunities for an A-orgy are unlimited. Vegetable eaters can gorge on all the vitamin A vegetables they want because carotene—previtamin A—is absolutely nontoxic. The worst thing that can happen if you overdose on carrots, collards, and dandelion greens is that your skin will turn a lovely yellow-orange. That's a sign you've had enough. In any event, all symptoms of vitamin A excess swiftly disappear when you go back to normal eating habits.

The most authoritative medical experts in the United States *do not* recommend vitamin A supplements for anyone over 4 years old. For those under 4, they have an interesting suggestion: 100,000 units of vitamin A every three months. That works out to 3 tablespoons of good old-fashioned cod liver oil on the first day of January, April, July, and October. Of course, that only applies to children who don't drink milk, since a quart of milk a day supplies 126,000 units every four months, and there you are!

While you can get more than enough vitamin A even from the simplest diet, most people *don't even have to eat* to get their dose of vitamin D.

How can that be?

It's simple. Everyone has his own personal vitamin D factory which can produce all he needs at no cost whatsoever. In fact, the only people who really run a big risk of vitamin D deficiency are black nuns working in Norway.

You see, the outer layer of your skin is transparent, and sunlight can penetrate to the layers below. The ultraviolet rays act on the cholesterol substances contained in the skin to form a chemical called *cholecalciferol,* otherwise known as *vitamin D$_3$.* (It's called D$_3$ because there are about ten known forms of the vitamin. Only two have practical importance: D$_3$ is one and D$_2$ is the other.) That homemade vitamin D passes directly into the bloodstream and is available for use by the body.

Vitamin D is an important vitamin—it regulates the calcium and phosphorus metabolism of the body. If you don't get enough D you might come down with rickets, a disease that causes softening of the bones. But it's very hard *not* to get enough vitamin D—unless you have black skin (which slows the production of vitamin D by sunlight), or wear the long sleeves and skirts of a nun's habit, or live in a country like Norway with scant sunshine. The dairy industry adds 400 international units of vitamin D per quart to milk sold in the United States. Actually that's not much trouble for the dairy industry, since all they have to do is flow the milk over ultraviolet lamps and the milk makes its *own* vitamin D.

How does that happen?

Well, milk contains cholesterol and related substances (specifically, a chemical called 7-dehydrocholesterol) just like human skin. Ultraviolet light converts some of the 7-dehydrocholesterol to vitamin D. So you can pay to have someone shine an expensive electric light on your milk—which you probably shouldn't be drinking anyway—or you can go outside and stand in the sun for a few minutes. You can do almost as well working in an office or factory in your shirt sleeves, since fluorescent lights produce ultraviolet too. Actually you don't need to do that, since the FDA, which is very keen on vitamins (even if it is about fifty years behind the times), admits that *no one over the age of 22 needs any extra vitamin D at all.* To make matters worse, of all the vitamins that line the drugstore shelves, vitamin D is the one that can make the most trouble for you if you take too much.

How much is too much?

As we mentioned, according to the FDA, for anyone over 22 years old, any amount of vitamin D—except what the skin manufactures and what you get in food—is *too much.* The vitamin is stored in body fat and can accumulate dangerously. An excess of vitamin D upsets calcium metabolism and can drain the calcium out of your bones and deposit it in your kidneys in the form of kidney stones. Babies are particularly sensitive to too much vitamin D— even 1000 units a day (only two and a half times the minimum) can make them very, very sick. When you put all the facts together, it seems obvious that no healthy persons should take vitamin D if they have a normal diet and get a few hours of sunshine a day. That applies particularly to babies, who can suffer serious and permanent damage from relatively small overdoses of the vitamin.*

Is it a good idea to take vitamin E?

Yes and no. It's nice to have some vitamin E in your diet. It's incredibly stupid to take vitamin E in tablets. Those are the facts. Now let's look at the fantasies.

Vitamin E has everything it takes to be a superstar—it's young, cheap, and sexy. And it got its first big start in life with sex. Back in 1922, an obscure trio of researchers locked some little rats up in cages and fed them a diet no rat would eat if he had any choice in the matter. Specifically the diet was lacking in grains, seeds, and all the other elements of a normal rat-diet. After a *couple of generations* of this sort of semistarvation, the male rats became sterile. (Humans would become sterile much faster on an equivalent diet.) Instantaneously vitamin E became famous as "the vitamin that cures sterility!" That statement wasn't true. A true statement was: "A diet deficient in many things, *including vitamin E,* produces sterility in caged rats." It is reasonable to assume—*although not necessarily correct*—that addition of vitamin E to that deficient rat-diet would cure *that* type of rat sterility. But *vitamin E is powerless to cure sterility from any other cause.* And sterility has never really been that big a problem—all it means is that a man who is sterile can't make a woman pregnant. That affects less than a fraction of 1 percent of American men.

On the other hand, impotence *is* a big problem. An impotent man can't perform sexually, because he either can't

* *Merck Manual of Diagnosis and Treatment,* 12th ed. Rahway, N.J., Merck & Co., 1972, p. 1065.

get an erection, keep an erection, or ejaculate at the right moment. A lot of men worry about things like that, and it didn't take the vitamin purveyors long to confuse "sterility" and "impotence" in the minds of vitamin buyers. Vitamin E then emerged as the poor man's aphrodisiac.* By verbal sleight-of-hand, what was supposed to be good for a grain-starved rat was peddled as good for a sex-starved man. Unfortunately there are a couple of problems.

What are the problems?

Well, there is one little detail to begin with: in the absence of severe disease, *a vitamin E deficiency just can't happen.* (And if someone is E deficient because of illness, he can swallow every vitamin E pill in the supermarket and it will only make him that much poorer.)

There is, however, one exception to that rule. Some American mothers who want the best for their young babies give them expensive imitation infant formulas which rob them of vitamin E. Those formulas that contain the new fashionable "polyunsaturated fats" have a tendency to rob any vitamin E available. Actually it's much better to choose another food supplement for your baby which contains a whopping 4 percent supersaturated animal fat and a big slug of vitamin E—along with every vitamin known and all the vitamins yet undiscovered. It's called *mother's milk*† (see Chapter XI).

Ironically the FDA only got around to declaring vitamin E "essential" in 1959, and they set the daily dose for infants at 4 units daily—or by coincidence just what most babies get from their mother's milk (or lose from the drugstore imitation). The adult "requirement" is supposed to be about 15 units a day, but don't panic if you haven't been taking vitamin E. You would have to eat 8760 consecutive meals without a speck of the vitamin to run the risk of a deficiency. (That means eight years without any E.) Considering that vitamin E is found abundantly in fats and

---

* Many vitamin E promotions hint broadly that E will cure impotence. That's a deliberate lie, but it sells vitamin E.
† *Merck Manual*, 12th ed., p. 1046.

oils, and that the typical American greasy diet is about *42 percent fat,* you get much more than you need. A table-spoon of corn oil, cottonseed oil, olive oil, peanut oil, or safflower oil provides plenty of the vitamin. It's also abundant in raw nuts, seeds, and soybeans.

But isn't it good to take vitamin E tablets just in case?

Just in case what? If you have high blood pressure or rheumatic heart disease, popping E pills can send you to your great reward—fast.*

If you're healthy, taking vitamin E supplements only picks your pocket. Let's do the calculations: One leading drug company advertises: "Our pills contain only the source of vitamin E closest to Nature. . . ." That would be vegetable oil, probably peanut or safflower oil. Each of their capsules contains 12 minims (a minim is a tiny unit of measure that druggists use). It takes 480 minims to make one ounce of oil. So a bottle of 500 capsules of vita-min E at an average cost of $50 a bottle gives you the ounce of peanut oil you could buy at the grocery store for about nine pennies. That outrageously overpriced bottle of cooking oil would supply you with about 37 years' worth of vitamin E—if you stopped eating altogether. Think of it this way, you've been buying plain old peanut oil at $160 a quart.

But if you have money to waste, don't stop at vitamin E pills. You can get E in cream, lotion, shampoo, bath oil, deodorant sticks, lipstick, eyesticks (whatever that is!), soap, dry power—and presumably for gourmets, you can get E mixed with garlic. But even then, it's not what it seems to be.

How come?

Vitamin E is composed of several chemical substances called *tocopherols.* There are seven of these, named after

---

* *Nutrition Almanac.* New York, McGraw-Hill, 1975, p. 51.

Greek letters: alpha, beta, delta, epsilon, eta, gamma, and zeta. The only tocopherol that can even *claim* any value is alpha. So those zingy full-page ads offer *all* the tocopherols —and then in very fine print tell you the truth: "No special claims are made for these substances since their presence is without any nutritional value whatsoever."

Not bad for peanut oil at $640 a gallon, eh? And suppose you take a few of these fabulously expensive little pills in the morning with your multivitamin pills and iron —what happens then? What happens is that the vitamin E interferes with the absorption of iron, and the iron interferes with the absorption of vitamin E, so you don't get the benefit of either one. Your $640 goes down the drain and you can even block the digestion of the iron and vitamin E in your daily diet. Does the label on your bottle of expensive vitamins warn you about that? If you think it does, check and see.*

Are there any more vitamins that are stored in fat?

Yes, there's one more. In addition to vitamins A, D, and E, vitamin K belongs to the fat-soluble group.

Vitamin K has the distinction of being about the only vitamin that is not hawked like breakfast cereal. That's not because the vitamin people wouldn't like to sell it to you. You can't buy it because you make it in abundance in your own large intestine. Humans produce all the K they need without any help from anyone. In serious disease there can be lack of K from malfunction of vital organs, but don't try to pop K pills in cases like that. You'd be buying a ticket to the cemetery.

In the next chapter we'll have a look at the vitamins that dissolve in water—the B-complex group and famous vitamin C. We may see that some of those wonderful claims also dissolve in water. Just turn the page.

---

* DiCyan, E., *Vitamins in Your Life*. New York, Simon and Schuster, 1972, p. 98.

CHAPTER II
Vitamins—Part Two

What are "B-complex" vitamins?

"B-complex" refers to all the water-soluble B vitamins—the most important of the group are the following:

B_1 or thiamine	Niacin or nicotinic acid
B_2 or riboflavin	Folic acid
B_6 or pyridoxine	Pantothenic acid
B_{12} or cyanocobalamin	Biotin

We've already had a short look at vitamin B_1 in relation to the work of the famous Dr. Funk. In healthy people, as is the case with all other vitamins, known and unknown, a deficiency of B_1 is virtually impossible unless someone eats a fad diet. Or to quote the medical textbook: "Primary (B_1) deficiency is confined to communities subsisting on polished rice." Check your cupboard to see if *you* subsist on white rice. As you will recall, polished or white rice has had all the vitamin B_1 removed in the process of refining.

In the United States and other industrial countries, beriberi is usually confined to alcoholics or, as they like to call themselves, "heavy drinkers." People who drink alcohol, besides all the other damage they do to their bodies, wipe out their stores of vitamin B_1. Drinking increases the requirement for B_1, reduces the intake of the vitamin, interferes with the absorption, and blocks the utilization. Aside from that it has no effect. So beriberi is a disease of drunks, colonizers and their victims, and folks who like nice fluffy white rice.

Incidentally, talking about "white," beautiful white refined sugar has exactly the same effect on B₁ as booze. It pushes vitamin-rich foods out of the diet, increases the need for the vitamin, robs B₁ from the body, and interferes with absorption. (*Unrefined* sugar doesn't cause any B₁ problems, since it brings its own B₁ with it.)

Another member of the "B" group is B₂ or riboflavin.

Is riboflavin an important vitamin?

If you don't get *any* it's important, but almost everyone gets more than he can use. The FDA thinks you should get exactly 1.7 thousandths of a gram a day—there being about 30 grams to an ounce. No one understands how they arrived at that odd figure, but there's plenty in nearly any kind of diet to supply that. Animal liver is particularly rich in riboflavin, but hundreds of other foods contain riboflavin and it's very very rare to see a deficiency.

Remember back in the good old days when milk came in bottles made of real glass? Remember those beautiful dark brown milk bottles that some companies used? They were to protect the riboflavin in your milk! When the milkman (remember the milkman?) used to put the milk on your front porch (in the days when people had front porches), the ultraviolet rays of the sun would rapidly destroy the riboflavin in the milk. But brown bottles blocked the ultraviolet rays and you got your vitamins. Those were the good old days.

One of the bad things about the good old days was pellagra.

What's pellagra?

A mere seventy years ago no one would have had to ask that question. At that time, pellagra was one of the major killing diseases in America. In the early years of the twentieth century there were more than *10,000 deaths a year* in the South alone. Another 200,000 men, women, and children were crippled by the disease every twelve months.

Pellagra has four stages, called the 4 "Ds": *dermatitis* (a reddish outbreak of the skin and mucous membranes), *dysentery* (severe uncontrollable diarrhea), *dementia* (deterioration of the ability to think), and finally *death*.

The official policy of the government and leading scientists was to ignore pellagra. After all, it only affected poor Southerners. But all those dead bodies finally became embarrassing, so the government authorized the Thompson-McFadden Commission to investigate. The commission carefully evaluated the diet of rural Southerners—those most susceptible to the disease—and drew their conclusions. Considering that these poor folks subsisted on cornmeal, grits, white flour, white rice, pork fat, white sugar, and sweet potatoes, the commission concluded that the disease that was killing them was the result of being bitten by a horsefly!

But couldn't they see the connection between the diet and the disease?

Not only couldn't they see the connection, but apparently they couldn't read. Nearly every medical book of the time told how Dr. Giuseppe Cerri cured an epidemic of pellagra in Milan in *1795* by changing the diet of the afflicted. As if that wasn't enough, the famous Dr. Roussel of France wrote a detailed thesis in 1845 establishing meat, milk, eggs, and fish as a cure for pellagra. But the Americans had to start all over again, just as if nothing had ever happened.

Getting rid of the horseflies didn't make any difference; the disease continued to rage. It took another commission to finally determine that pellagra in the American South was the same as pellagra in Italy and pellagra in France. And the cure was the same—a tiny improvement in the diet.

When it was reestablished that a dietary deficiency

caused pellagra, a gigantic race began to find a vitamin that could be sold at immense profits to prevent and cure the disease. Finally in 1937 a drug called *nicotinic acid* was isolated from animal livers and found to be substantially effective in preventing pellagra. That's when the famous Dr. Funk comes back into the picture.

What did he have to do with nicotinic acid?

He discovered it—way back in 1911, at least twenty-six years before anyone else in the world suspected that it even existed. Unfortunately he didn't have Dr. Eijkman's Javanese houseboy to tell him the significance of his discovery, so he just poured it down the sink. That's right, after painstakingly isolating this elusive chemical, he simply threw it away because he didn't know what to do with it. Another achievement in the exciting panorama of vitamin research!

But twenty-six years later, the tireless vitamin chemists finally repeated Funk's work and succeeded in making synthetic nicotinic acid. The product now sells for about $4 a pound wholesale. In a little brown jar at the drugstore in the form of white pills it runs about $612 a pound. Not bad for something you can get free while you're eating lunch.

In reality the entire epidemic of pellagra could have been avoided, tens of thousands of lives could have been saved, and million of cases of disability could have been avoided for *peanuts*.

You mean that nicotinic acid could have been made in the laboratory at lower cost?

No, I mean that a handful of peanuts every other day or so would have prevented the deadly epidemic of pellagra. The humble little goober that grows all over the South contains 17.2 milligrams of nicotinic acid in each 3½ ounce serving. The slightly hysterical FDA recommends 18 milligrams a day of nicotinic acid for men, 13 milligrams for women (sexism!), and less for children. For the poor people in the cities in those days it was even easier. Butchers used to give liver away free for dog food —it wasn't considered fit for human consumption. One serving of hog liver (the cheapest kind) contains about 22 milligrams of nicotinic acid.

What's the difference between niacin and nicotinic acid?

Public relations. The correct chemical name for the substance is *nicotinic acid,* but when they first started selling it for $612 a pound in pills, sales were slow. People thought they were being sold something awful like nicotine, so the merchandisers found a new name. They took the *ni* from "nicotinic," the *ac* from "acid," and the *in* from "vitamin," to get the new name, *niacin.* Sales picked up. Niacin, nicotinic acid, niacinamide, nicotinamide are all basically the same thing. If nicotinic acid had been discovered today, Madison Avenue wouldn't have settled for such a prosaic name as *niacin.* They would have called it "Aphrodite Super-Formula F-29" and sold it in fluorescent purple capsules scented with genuine imitation musk oil. .

Then niacin is the absolute cure for pellagra?

Yes and no. When the chemists begin to fiddle with the food we eat, things can get bad very quickly. The diet of the poor Southerners was chemically manipulated: white flour, white cornmeal, refined corn grits, white sugar, white rice. All these substances were chemically raped before they were sold to the unsuspecting consumer. Then the chemists did it again by offering to sell them niacin to undo the harm they had inflicted in the first place. But if you eat a crummy diet and take niacin, you can *still* get pellagra.

How can that be?

Because, as it turns out, pellagra is a disease of *multiple* vitamin deficiencies. Niacin is the most important cause, but lack of thiamine, riboflavin, and another substance, pyridoxine (vitamin B_6), also plays a role.

All that trouble and suffering can be avoided by getting your vitamins in a perfectly balanced combination—not pills from the supermarket but fresh, natural, wholesome foods, where vitamins come from in the first place. And it's so easy. It's true that pellagra can be prevented by peanuts, but you don't even need them. If those folks had just eaten pumpkin seeds, squash seeds, or even crunched the seeds of the watermelons all of them ate, pellagra never would have happened.

As a matter of fact, you don't even have to consume any niacin at all to avoid pellagra.

But didn't you just finish saying that lack of niacin causes pellagra?

That's right. But if your diet includes a common essential amino acid called *tryptophan,* all your niacin worries are over, because your body has the capacity to automatically convert *tryptophan into niacin.* Since tryptophan is found in thousands of diverse foods, it makes it doubly foolish to take niacin supplements. Look at an example: about 5 ounces of baked flounder supplies 450 milligrams of tryptophan, which the body can convert into about 7.5 milligrams of niacin. That's about half the FDA recommended daily allowance—which is far more than any person actually needs to avoid a deficiency. (The FDA characteristically overestimates the actual vitamin requirements of human beings—perhaps out of consideration for vitamin manufacturers?) For every 60 milligrams of tryptophan you consume, your own little vitamin factory turns out 1 milligram of niacin. What more could you ask?

Are there any other important B-complex vitamins?

There are a few. Vitamin B6 is worth mentioning, as an example of how to pay more to get less. This vitamin is really composed of three separate substances: pyridoxine, pyridoxinal, and pyridoxamine, although it is usually called simply *pyridoxine*. The overstated FDA recommended requirement is only 2 milligrams, and it's almost impossible to avoid soaking that much up from your daily diet, since the vitamin is found in all meat, whole wheat products, and thousands of other everyday foods.

However, a certain number of American mothers, at great expense, succeeded in giving their infants a deficiency of B6. You see, these days it's fashionable to feed your baby artificial milk instead of the real kind. Artificial milk has a picture of a smiling baby on the can, is advertised in all the best magazines, and costs a lot of money. Therefore, it must be good! Nobody takes TV spots on the eleven o'clock news to advertise breast milk, do they? But the inferior artificial milks—known as "infant formula"—were deficient in vitamin B6, and the manufacturers added artificial B6 to the product—about one sixteenth of a cent's worth, more or less. Then they sterilized the mixture and destroyed all the B6. The babies who drank the stuff soon developed a full-blown B6 deficiency complete with convulsions and all the rest.* The "disadvantaged" kids who drink mother's milk just keep growing.

But it was pantothenic acid that provided the biggest challenge to the merchandisers of vitamins.

Why was that?

Because this, of all vitamins, is found in *all living cells* —that's how it got its name. The *pan* in pantothenic stands for "occurring everywhere." For all practical purposes, anyone who eats food is forever safe from a deficiency of pantothenic acid. A deficiency has never been found in a

---

* *Merck Manual*, 12th ed., p. 1055.

normal human being, and there is no reliable way to even detect a deficiency. But that never stopped a dedicated vitamin company. Years of experiments finally produced a strange chemical called omega-methyl pantothenic acid; that was the turning point. By feeding this poison to paid volunteers it was possible to burn up all the pantothenic acid in their bodies and actually produce a deficiency of pantothenic acid! The FDA then did their part and declared pantothenic acid essential and concocted a Recommended Daily Allowance of 10 milligrams. The vitamin companies began including it in their formulas, and a whole new industry was born. But they do it in a funny way—the usual vitamin formula includes about 120 millionths of a gram, or a mere fraction of the just-as-stupid FDA recommended allowance. They put it there just to have the name on the label, but if you pay one cent a tablet for 120 micrograms of pantothenic acid, you are shelling out $40,000 a pound for a vitamin that you couldn't keep out of your diet if you tried. And they say there's no profit in the vitamin business?

Are there any other vitamins like that?

You mean expensive little names tacked onto pills that nobody needs to take? Yes, there are a few more laughable examples. Take biotin, for example. In the 50,000-year history of man, nobody has ever seen a naturally occurring case of biotin deficiency. Finally the hardworking scientists fed some poor fellow—get this—nothing but egg whites! The FDA obligingly cranked out a daily allowance for biotin: three tenths of a milligram a day. If you're going to try to make it on only egg whites—oh, yes, those have to be *raw* egg whites—better take your biotin tabs. They will run you about $16,000 a pound at a penny a tablet for your daily ration—a bargain, you must admit, in comparison to pantothenic acid. Actually, like pantothenic acid, it's hard to find a food that doesn't contain some biotin.

And one final detail that they forget to put on the label of that bottle of vitamins: biotin is manufactured within your body so you have all you need all the time—*free*. Whoever said the vitamin sellers were cynical?

But aren't some of the B vitamins important?

They're all important—that's why they're in food. But just because a nutrient is important doesn't mean you have to run out and spend $40,000 a pound to buy it in the form of pills. Folic acid is a good example. A deficiency of that vitamin causes a severe kind of anemia—an anemia that all the patent-medicine "iron tonics" peddled on television won't touch. But like the other vitamins, it's almost impossible to get a deficiency if you just eat a reasonable diet. The name of folic acid comes from the Latin word *folia*, which means "leaves." Green leafy vegetables, most meats, fresh fruits, whole grains, all provide plenty of folic acid. But there are two situations where folic acid can be a problem.

Pregnant women on a diet of modern "convenience" foods may not get enough folic acid, since it is destroyed by heating and processing. The drug companies have convinced doctors that the solution is to give these victims of mass malnutrition pills of folic acid. A smarter way is for pregnant women (and everyone else) to simply eat fresh natural food—and forget the pills. Millions of women give birth to millions of normal healthy babies all over the world without popping a single pill. They must be doing something right.

Theoretically, during pregnancy the body's requirement for folic acid doubles. That means instead of the 400 micrograms a day recommended by the FDA, a pregnant woman theoretically needs 800 micrograms daily. (Remember now that a microgram is one millionth of a gram, and a gram is about one thirtieth of an ounce. It's not a lot of folic acid any way you look at it.) All the pregnant lady has to do is eat one ounce of fried beef liver once in a while. That ounce gives her about 62.5 milligrams of folic acid, or 78 times her expanded daily requirement. Besides, folic acid is not nearly as soluble in water as the other B vitamins and

29

can be stored in the liver. You don't have to eat it *every* day.

At the other extreme are women who don't want to be pregnant, the ones who take birth-control pills. Those potentially deadly hormone combinations deplete folic acid stores and can cause severe anemia. The solution is not to take folic acid but to use a less dangerous means of contraception. And folic acid, of all the vitamins that you can buy in the supermarket, is the one that can be the most deadly.

How can it be deadly?

There is a serious disease called *pernicious anemia* related to a lack of another vitamin, vitamin B_{12}. Pernicious anemia is a dangerous disease; it can cause severe weight loss, paralysis, psychosis, and total disability in its final stages. However, the early symptoms are relatively mild: weakness, fatigue, palpitations. In the early stages, victims tend to read those sensational vitamin ads and start popping folic acid pills from their local drugstore. What happens next can be disastrous.

They start to feel worse?

No, they start to feel *better*. Folic acid relieves the *superficial* symptoms of pernicious anemia while the destruction of the brain and spinal cord continues unchecked. Months later, when the victim is permanently paralyzed, it becomes obvious that gulping folic acid wasn't such a good idea.

But the FDA has a solution for that problem too. It prohibits the sale without prescription of folic acid pills that contain more than 400 micrograms of the substance. The reasoning is that 400 micrograms a day isn't enough to cover up the mild symptoms of pernicious anemia so patients won't be lulled into thinking they have cured themselves from the drugstore. A brilliant idea from the FDA! But what about the people who take two or three folic acid tablets a day? They will succeed in masking their symptoms. Well, FDA, back to the drawing board.

Folic acid is expensive too—when you buy it by the pill. Assuming a retail price of one cent a tablet—if you find it that cheap—you get about 60 micrograms in each pill and not the FDA limit of 400 micrograms. That will set you back about $80,000 a pound. Before you rush out, try frying a little liver. Even if you don't like the taste, think of the money you'll save. And you'll never have to worry about masking a dread disease like pernicious anemia.

How do you prevent pernicious anemia?

You can't.* Pernicious anemia is the result of a deficiency of vitamin B_{12}, but taking all the B_{12} in the world won't prevent you from getting the disease since it is caused by a built-in defect in the way a person's body absorbs the vitamin. Actually the situation is unique among vitamins, since there are two "factors" involved for B_{12} utilization. One is the *extrinsic factor,* or vitamin B_{12} itself. The other is the *intrinsic factor,* or a certain substance that allows B_{12} to pass through the wall of the stomach or intestine. People who get pernicious anemia are those who just don't have the intrinsic factor in their digestive juices. No matter how many B_{12} pills they swallow, they just can't absorb the vitamin.

Incidentally, there is also a rare cause of B_{12} deficiency which doesn't really qualify as pernicious anemia. People who eat raw fish can get a fish tapeworm called *Diphyllobothrium,* which lives in the intestine and eats all the B_{12} before it can get to the victim. That's as bad as a brother-in-law who sits in your favorite chair, smokes your best cigars, and drinks your best whiskey.

---

* Since pernicious anemia is defined as absence of the intrinsic factor and is genetically determined, it cannot be "prevented," although a patient can be kept in remission by adequate medical treatment.

What's the treatment for pernicious anemia?

See your doctor, not your vitamin salesman. The doctor will confirm the diagnosis and give you tiny injections of vitamin B_{12} to clear up your symptoms. And *tiny* is the word—in the beginning you'll probably get 100 millionths of a gram per week and then the same microscopic dose every month for a total dose of 1200 millionths of a gram per year! Injections may seem like a nuisance, but it was worse the other way.

What was the "other way"?

Before B_{12} was available in injection form, victims of pernicious anemia had to get their missing intrinsic and extrinsic factors from its original source. That meant they had to eat *raw* liver at least once a day—and not just a nibble. Most of them ate it gladly, although they didn't exactly wolf it down. Those who didn't eat their liver weren't around very long.

But isn't it a good idea to take vitamin B_{12} just in case?

It's not a matter of "just in case." Of course it's a good idea to take vitamin B_{12}. But that's not a problem. The problem is how can anyone *avoid* taking vitamin B_{12}? The chemical is in virtually every food of animal origin, and even though it is water-soluble, it takes a long time for symptoms of deficiency to appear after you stop all intake of B_{12}. The FDA Recommended Daily Allowance is a whopping 6 micrograms a day, which is an excellent example of the way the FDA encourages overconsumption of expensive and unnecessary vitamins. Everybody thinks— or used to think—"if the government recommends it, then it must be good." Let's see. Six micrograms a day of B_{12} adds up to 186 micrograms a month of an expensive vitamin. If you had a life-threatening deficiency of the chemical and *were not absorbing any at all from your diet*, your doctor would only give you 100 micrograms a month. But your government encourages you to take almost twice as much as the victims of pernicious anemia—who really need it!

But what about people who don't eat any B_{12} at all? Don't they need to take B_{12} pills?

That's what they'd like you to believe. Some prominent nutritionists, who should know better, tell us that it is absolutely essential to eat meat to avoid a "dangerous" deficiency of B_{12}. (By coincidence some of these same "experts" are paid consultants to the powerful meat producers' associations.) The dumbest thing they say is that vegetarians are living on borrowed time because they can't get any B_{12} from a vegetarian diet. That news will come as a surprise to 500,000,000 Hindus, most of whom don't eat any meat or animal products at all from the moment they are born until the moment they die (with the exception of mother's milk for a while). The Hindu religion has been around for over 10,000 years, or about 98 centuries longer than "modern American medicine." Deficiencies of B_{12} are virtually unknown among these vegetarians, and they miss out on a few other little things too, like cancer of the colon, heart attacks, diabetes, and other "signs of progress."

There are several possible explanations that seem reasonable. First, people who don't gorge on meat develop the ability to recycle their vitamin B_{12} instead of urinating it all away. Second, some vegetables do contain small amounts of B_{12}. Third, vegetarians possibly develop the ability to produce their own B_{12} from intestinal fermentation, like sheep and some other animals.

Of course, you wouldn't expect anything with a name like "B_{12}" to be cheap, would you? After all double-digit vitamins run high. A popular formula of B_{12} gives you 5 micrograms for two cents a tablet. That figures out to just about *$2 million a pound*. Don't you feel sorry for those folks who have to settle for a diamond mine instead of a vitamin pill factory? So forget about all those dire threats

33

of the play-for-pay nutritional experts—just ask yourself how come they don't look so healthy themselves.

Are there any other B vitamins?

There sure are, but get ready for some laughs. The pill pushers have reached way out into left field for some of them. Vitamin B_{13} is a good example. Made from sour milk, it is not yet available in the United States, unless, of course, you sip a little sour milk. (Vitamin sellers don't recommend that—it's not good for business.) No one has figured out how much you need of this new addition to the vitamin alphabet, or whether you even need it at all, but that never stopped big names like vitamin E back in the early days.

Another "B" is choline. No one knows the daily requirement of choline, or *if there is a daily requirement*. Choline will never make it big, since it is manufactured every day right in your own body.

Inositol is in the same boat as choline. For lack of any better information, vitamin sellers recommend you take the same amount of inositol pills as you take choline pills. I agree wholeheartedly with that suggestion, provided you aren't taking any choline to begin with.

Now we come to the most interesting B vitamin of all: vitamin B_{17}, also known as Laetrile or amygdalin. Everyone has read the exciting stories of midnight raids by the dauntless men of the FDA to arrest desperate criminals who sell this harmless extract of apricot kernels.

Why do they arrest them?

Because some chemists and a certain number of reputable physicians believe that Laetrile can cure or at least arrest cancer. The substance that makes up Laetrile is composed of two molecules of sugar, one molecule of benzaldehyde, and one molecule of cyanide. You can get your dose of amygdalin—complete with cyanide—from the little nut inside the seed of apricots, peaches, cherries, plums, and other similar fruits. "For your safety and comfort . . . ," as they say when the airlines bully the passengers, the FDA forbids the sale of a substance that might cure cancer. It allows the sale of many substances that *produce* cancer. (A list includes carcinogenic food coloring, PCB, diethylstilbestrol, and at least 100 other hazardous chemicals. See the appropriate chapters for details.)

But isn't cyanide a poison?

It sure is, if you take enough of it. But then so is table salt, MSG, caffeine, and aspirin in excessive quantities. Cyanide is normally found in small amounts in more than 2000 commonly consumed foods; you've probably had some already today, so don't worry about it.

But is vitamin B₁₇ any good as a cancer cure?

Who knows? There are a couple of interesting things about B₁₇. First, a lot of distinguished doctors think it produces results. Second, it's harmless. Third, it is used every day to treat cancer patients in about 20 other countries, including such medically advanced nations as Germany, Italy, Belgium, and Canada. Fourth, about 7000 years ago, the ancient Chinese got pretty good results using the same treatment for cancer: apricot kernels. Fifth, it is very cheap, by comparison. (Radical cancer surgery can set you back $50,000 if you include all the costs such as time lost from work.)

The one possibility that strikes fear into the hearts of cancer specialists is that people might start treating themselves for cancer. Of course, if vitamin B₁₇ is given a fair trial as a prescription drug, we'll quickly find out one way or the other. Strangely enough, in those 20 countries and even in the United States there are quite a few people who *think* they've been cured of cancer by B₁₇. Truthfully, *I don't know if it works or not*. The FDA doesn't know either. It wouldn't hurt anyone to find out, would it?

35

Are there any other B vitamins that are important?

A couple. Take PABA, for instance. Its full name is *para-aminobenzoic acid,* and it's in many of the multiple vitamins you can buy at the supermarket. No one knows how much you need, you make more than enough every day in your own body, and it's sheer madness to take even a single tablet. But it's smart to rub PABA on your skin if you want to avoid a sunburn. In a 5 percent concentration, it is one of the best sunscreens known.

The last on the list is vitamin B15, also known as *pangamic acid.* About the only thing B15 has going for it is that you won't find it in many supermarket vitamin pills—yet.

But don't vitamins have any medical qualities?

Of course they do. Vitamins are chemical substances, and like all chemicals in large enough amounts they can have significant effects on the human body. Think of it this way—the amount of a vitamin required to prevent the symptoms of a vitamin deficiency can be measured in thousandths or even millionths of a gram. Those are the amounts you easily obtain in the several pounds of food you eat every day—provided you eat decent unprocessed food.

There is also a separate branch of medicine called *megavitamin therapy* where vitamins are given in massive doses —thousands of times the actual daily requirement—to treat alcoholism, senility, mental illnesses, and hypoglycemia. While all the returns aren't in, megavitamin therapy has one thing going for it: the medical establishment is against it. The powers-that-be in medicine have been against every major medical improvement in the past 500 years, including anesthesia, vaccination, sterile surgery, and the high-fiber diet.

There is a legitimate place for vitamins in the medical treatment of certain diseases. These include vitamin K in some coagulation problems, vitamin B12 in pernicious anemia, and vitamin D in certain disorders of the parathyroid gland.

But trying to cure "tiredness," "lack of pep," sexual impotence, and a thousand other self-diagnosed conditions by popping commercial vitamins is sheer madness. Instead of throwing away hundreds of millions of dollars every year on vitamins in the form of pills that they can get for nothing in the form of breakfast, lunch, and supper, Americans should save their money. When they have enough, they can just invite a friend over to dinner. Believe me, it's a better investment.

CHAPTER III
Vitamins—Part Three

Is vitamin C really as important as all those articles say it is?

Probably not. Vitamin C is just another of the thousand or so chemicals your body needs to function well. The whole game of vitamin merchandising seems to be something like this: select a nice everyday plain-jane chemical, spin a romantic story about it, gather a few made-to-order scientific articles about how vital it is, and then sell it for about 10,000 times what it costs you. Check this example:

"Microcrystalline vitamin B_4, brought to you from deep within mysterious eastern mountains. A pure white glittering powder, it holds within it *the secret of all life*. Every cell of your body cries out for B_4; it is absolutely essential for your existence. Scientists have proved that a deficiency of this life-giving factor can be responsible for loss of memory, disturbed thinking, heart palpitations, stomach pains, poor digestion, and many other everyday problems. Serious deficiencies can cause death! Available in mini-tablets and a form you can't resist: exclusive instant-dissolving flavor crystals to sprinkle on your food. Protect your health today. Get vitamin B_4 in the handy gourmet shaker-pack!"

Before you rush out and get your "gourmet shaker-pack" of vitamin B_4, *think*. Vitamin B_4 is nothing more than good old sodium chloride, otherwise known as table salt. But the vitamin hustlers haven't told you any outright lies.

It's dug from "deep within mountains"—salt mines. Every cell of your body does need salt; lack of salt can make you sick, and if you lose enough salt you will die. You probably can't resist those "instant-dissolving flavor crystals" to sprinkle on your food, but when you buy them ask for "salt" at about twenty-five cents a pound, not "vitamin B_4," which will run about $100 a pound when someone gets around to promoting it.

Isn't that an exaggerated price?

It certainly is, but that's what they're charging for "vitamins" these days. Let's examine the story of vitamin C and let's calculate how much *that* costs a pound. You'll be fascinated.

What is "The Vitamin C Story"?

It is a tale full of intrigue, heroism, genius, and stupidity —mostly stupidity. Everyone who has studied history is familiar with the epidemics of scurvy that ravaged sailors in the sixteenth, seventeenth, and eighteenth centuries. Famous expeditions like those of Vasco da Gama, Magellan, and Jacques Cartier all suffered terribly from scurvy. But how about the Chinese navigators who stayed at sea for months at a time, far from their morning orange juice? What about the Vikings who crossed and recrossed the Atlantic long before Columbus? Why didn't they suffer death and crippling from scurvy?

Well, why didn't they get scurvy?

Let's see what scurvy's all about. Most species of animals synthesize vitamin C within their own bodies—they never need even a millimicrogram of the chemical from the outside. There are a few unfortunate exceptions, including man, gorillas, monkeys, guinea pigs, the bulbul bird, and the fruit-eating bat. (That's why he eats fruit.) None of the other so-called "wild" animals ever get deficiencies of C— unless they are put in cages and fed man-food. But humans, if they are deprived of vitamin C for long periods of time —three months to a year—may develop the symptoms of scurvy. These include badly swollen gums, loss of teeth, and defects in wound healing. Ultimately death occurs. So scurvy is a bad disease, but it doesn't strike you down if you forget to drink your orange juice for three days in a row. It takes almost total deprivation of vitamin C in any form for extended periods. Any time during the latent period of up to a year, it can be prevented or reversed by relatively small doses of C. The only people who really get scurvy these days in the United States are those who rigidly follow the so-called macrobiotic diet. They live almost exclusively on brown rice, which is nice but is hardly a well-balanced menu.

But what about those poor sailors who died of scurvy?

They were victims of greed and stupidity—nothing else. In those days seamen were fed a diet of salt fish, salt beef, and crackers made from rye flour. There wasn't an ounce of vitamin C in a ton of that stuff. If you read the history books carefully, you'll find that it was mostly the common sailors who got scurvy—not the officers. The sailors were generally fed according to contract; a private firm agreed to provision the ship for the voyage for a fixed sum—and the cheaper the food, the greater their profit. The officers had a few luxuries like potatoes, and that made the difference. Stupidity played a role as well. Rarely were the ships at sea as long as three months without landing—and if the sailors had only eaten fresh fruits and vegetables when they went ashore, they would have aborted the attacks of scurvy.

The Vikings had a simpler solution: they just ate sauerkraut.

Sauerkraut?

Sure. Sauerkraut has 64 milligrams of vitamin C per pound, more than enough to prevent scurvy. The Chinese did even better; they grew their own bean sprouts on long voyages: 86 milligrams of vitamin C per pound. Even the FDA, which always overestimates vitamin requirements, only pushes for 45 milligrams a day.

Finally, about 1600, lemon juice was introduced into the British Navy to prevent scurvy. It produced almost miraculous results, but then, to save money, they stopped using it and scurvy broke out again. It wasn't until about 1750 that lemon juice was reintroduced. And in some cases sailors who drank lemon juice still came down with scurvy!

But how could that be?

Because the sailors were so stupid that they *boiled* the lemon juice to make it "pure." In the process, the heat destroyed all the vitamin C in the juice and they got scurvy. But they were ignorant, uneducated sailors in the middle of the eighteenth century. No one could be that dumb—with one exception.

What exception was that?

The pediatricians of America who single-handedly inflicted a deadly epidemic of scurvy on the infants of the United States some eighty years ago! These brilliant medical specialists warned mothers to vigorously boil the milk they gave their infants. Fearfully the mothers complied, cooked away the vitamin C, and gave their helpless babies scurvy.*

Fortunately these days no one has to worry about destroying the vitamin C in their children's food—the food-

---

* Collective investigation of infantile scurvy in North America. *Journal of the American Pediatric Society*, 1898.

processing industry does it for you. Look at some of the figures:

A 3½ ounce portion of raw carrots contains 8 milligrams of vitamin C. By the time they get into a can, 6 mg of C have been cooked away, leaving a bare 2 mg. You have been cheated out of 75 percent of your vitamin C, and the price has gone up in the process. Freezing food does about the same. Fresh broccoli has 90 mg of C per 3½ ounce serving. Frozen broccoli has only 57 mg, a loss of about 37 percent—but the price doesn't go *down* 37 percent.

Apples are another good example. Raw apples contain 7 mg of vitamin C in 3½ ounces. By the time they get into applesauce, the vitamin C has almost vanished. They've heated away 6 of the 7 mg, leaving 1 lonesome milligram for a loss of 85 percent of the C content. The processors do a better job on baby applesauce. It only contains what they call a "trace" of vitamin C. Try and find it.

But if you really want to see something, take a look at orange juice.

What about orange juice?

Kindly remove your hat when you speak about orange juice for this is the sacred liquid to 220 million Americans. By a miracle of advertising, the orange growers of the United States have convinced us that eating oranges and drinking orange juice are sensible ways of getting vitamin C and *curing colds*. (More about that last part later.) They are wrong for telling us that, and we are wrong for believing it! Penny for penny and milligram for milligram, oranges and orange juice are an awful source of vitamin C.

If you want larger amounts of vitamin C at lower cost than orange juice, try any of the following: broccoli, Brussels sprouts, collards, turnip greens, mustard greens, and red cabbage. Hot peppers have 400 percent more vitamin C than the orangiest orange. Tomatoes, spinach, asparagus, liver, and ham are excellent sources of C. Even the lowly baked potato (skin included) contains a nice shot of C. But no one thinks of these foods as packed with vitamin

C, probably because so far no sexy chick has gone on TV to do thirty-second commercials for, say, Brussels sprouts. Think of it:

(Camera moves in slowly on girl singer, concentrating on her well-filled low-cut blouse.) Raising arms over her head, she sings loudly:

"It's gonna be a good day! So let's get out and shout, eat a BRUSSELS SPROUT! It's gonna be a good day!"

Announcer (speaks sincerely): "So, friends, to get the full benefit of vitamin C and really come alive, every day should start out with a Brussels sprout! Hallelujah!"

(Ends with close-up of singer's mammary glands.)

If you like the taste of orange juice, drink it, but don't pay too much attention to the claims on the label.

What about the claims on the label?

For a report on *that,* let's check the *Wall Street Journal,* which no one could ever accuse of being biased toward the consumer. In the issue of June 16, 1976, on page 25, the headline reads:

CARTON ORANGE JUICE IS FOUND
LACKING IN ACTIVE VITAMIN C

That doesn't sound too good, does it? Well, hang on for the rest. Two researchers at the Mt. Sinai School of Medicine of the City University of New York did what someone should have done long ago. They went around the corner to the grocery store, bought some orange juice, and analyzed it to see how much vitamin C it actually contained. Boy, were they surprised! This is what they found (according to the *Wall Street Journal*):

Freshly squeezed orange juice contained about 80 mg per 100 cc (or about 3½ ounces) of active vitamin C. Frozen juice had about the same. However, orange juice that comes in cartons had (in some cases) about *half the active vitamin C content of fresh or frozen juice,* although they weren't selling the product at half the price. However, an executive for a major juice company sneered: "We

44

don't speculate on the form (active or inactive) that the vitamin C is in." Why should they? They don't buy the stuff, they sell it.

What do you have to do to be sure to get enough vitamin C?

Nothing. Even the super-junky average American diet has more vitamin C than you need. Lettuce, potato chips, peas, cole slaw, and even plain old ketchup contain big slugs of C. About the only way to get scurvy is to restrict your diet to only one C-deficient food, like the brown rice of the "Zen macrobiotic diet," which doesn't have that much to do with Zen. People in supposedly primitive countries don't get scurvy because they never get the chance to sink their teeth into all those garbagey processed foods. But if you're really determined to get extra vitamin C, there's a cheap, easy way to do it: eat a green pepper! Ounce for ounce, raw green peppers have twice the vitamin C content of orange juice.

What about vitamin C and the common cold?

Oh, yes. Isn't that exciting? A man says that if you take 2 or 3 or 4 grams of vitamin C a day, it will cure your cold or prevent you from getting a cold. I remember what my old professor of medicine used to tell us when we studied viral diseases: "Gentlemen, a cold normally clears up by itself in seven days. An injection of penicillin will always cure a cold within a week." So you get a cold, take vitamin C, you get over the cold, and the C gets the credit. Not bad for the folks who sell vitamin C. Assume that each of, say, 150 million people get two colds a year. Calculate that only half can be coaxed to take 4 of the 500 mg vitamin C tablets daily—that's 2 grams a day for 5 days. The final count is 3 billion tablets a year. At a retail cost of only two cents a tablet, the bill is a mere $60 million a year. If anybody had any proof that vitamin C really cured a cold it *might* be worth it.

45

But doesn't vitamin C also *prevent* colds?

How would anyone know? All those exciting studies about people who take massive doses of vitamin C having fewer colds don't make much sense. Let's say you had four colds last year without taking vitamin C. This year you took big doses of vitamin C and only had three colds. To really prove the vitamin reduced the number of colds you had, you would actually have to live this year over again without taking the vitamin to see if you had more colds without C. Maybe this year was just a better year for colds, and maybe if you didn't take C you would've only had two colds. Besides, it just isn't a big deal. A cold is a nonfatal self-limiting disease which is socially useful. Eighty-four percent of all colds occur on Fridays and Mondays and give you an excuse for a long weekend. And consider for a moment the cost of taking vitamin C. One nationally advertised C tablet gives you 100 mg of C for two cents a tablet. That works out to a mere $100 per pound. You can get twice as much vitamin C (plus a lot of other vitamins) in a completely natural form in one small green pepper.

Don't babies need vitamin C?

Sure they do; they're no different from anyone else. Breast-feeding is the best way to give an infant vitamin C —and everything else it needs. Breast milk supplies 5 milligrams of C in about 3½ ounces. That's fine for a baby. Instead of buying expensive vitamin concoctions, you can give your baby a few teaspoons of orange juice (unboiled —remember the British sailors!) every morning or tomato juice in somewhat larger quantities. Both should be freshly squeezed. (Just put the tomato in the blender and strain the juice.) Remember, no one can prepare, package and provide for the assimilation of those vitamins better than the Being who created us all.

Even though a person may not need all those extra vitamin pills, what if he feels better after he takes them?

That's fine. The Romans even had a word for it: *placebo,* which means "I please." In English, a placebo is a medicine, usually a nice-looking little pill, that has no physical effect but usually makes the patient feel better just because he's taking *something.* Imported placebos always work better than the domestic kind, and expensive placebos in blue glass jars are the best of all. Virtually all vitamin pills are placebos. They contain tiny amounts of vitamins and massive proportions of cheap stuff like cornstarch, refined sugar, and other fillers. The interesting thing is that placebos do make a certain number of people feel better.

Researchers often use what is called the *double-blind* method in testing a new drug. They give half of a group, say 50 people, the real drug under study. They give another 50 people a drug that *appears identical* but contains only cornstarch. (That's the single-blind part of the experiment.) If they are testing a new drug against arthritis, let's say, usually 30 people in the group getting the real drug will feel better. But about 20 people with joint pains get relief from pretty pills containing cornstarch! It's certainly logical, since every part of the body, including the joints, is attached directly to the mind—and the mind has the final say in everything.

What's the "double-blind" part of the experiment?

The doctors who are administering the medicine aren't told which pills are which or which group is getting the real medicine. The idea is that if they knew, they would unconsciously influence the patients to get better. And, of course, it happens that way. If the doctor gives you a pill and says, "This will make you feel better before lunch-time," he has already given you a big shove toward health. Now look at the vitamin ads and see what they say:

"Vitamin E potency to work for a more radiant lovelier skin!"

"Vitamin C—C-Power at its total best!"

"Brewers' Yeast plus B_{12} has an impressive 500 micrograms per pound of vitamin B_{12}!"

"Super-Action for nutritional peace of mind! Provides a potent supply of essential nutrients to help protect against vitamin deficiencies!'

Maybe you don't even have to take those expensive vitamins—just read the ads every morning.

Are natural vitamins better than synthetic?

Natural vitamins are better for natural people. When scientists succeed in manufacturing people in the laboratory, then they should feed them the vitamins they make in the laboratory. A natural vitamin (or mineral) is one that you consume in food as part of your daily diet. A synthetic or artificial vitamin is one that is made in a chemical laboratory from chemicals found there. It may have a similar chemical composition to the real thing and even a *similar* effect, but *it is not the same*. It's not the same because it is made from different ingredients than the naturally occurring vitamin, and it is not consumed with the same background of other food elements that the natural vitamins are.

Can you give an example?

Certainly. Let's take oranges. The vitamin C you get from a pill is ascorbic acid, cooked up in a chemical lab. You take it by itself or with whatever you may happen to be eating—a potato, a cup of coffee, a cough drop. The vitamin C in an orange is truly natural vitamin C, and every bite of the orange carries, along with vitamin C, in an inseparable form, the following nutrients: calcium, phosphorus, iron, sodium, potassium, vitamin A, thiamine, riboflavin, and niacin—*plus many more still undiscovered nutrients.*

48

Beyond that, it is a well-known principle in nutrition that the availability (to the body) of important food substances often depends on the *simultaneous presence* of other food elements. Maybe vitamin C doesn't really work for you unless it is taken with the precisely correct amount of nine other substances—only three of which have been discovered so far. You'll never know if you keep popping pills, will you?

But don't vitamin preparations contain natural vitamins?

How could they? They may be made from *natural* sources, but by the time they are baked, boiled, roasted, toasted, dried, extracted with chemical solvents, and pushed into little pills with cornstarch, they have forgotten where they came from. One typical example is "natural" vitamin A tablets made from carrot oil, of all things. The ad says:

"Capsulated vitamin A from the finest grown carrots! Select carrots, deep-rooted, grown in rich soil, are the only source for this potent vitamin A!"

Those people buy carrot *seeds*, mash them up, use a chemical to extract the carrot oil, and then "capsulate" it. (That means pushing it into capsules, by the way.) The carrot oil you buy at two cents a capsule is about as natural as a cornflake. The one thing missing from the ad is an explanation of why you should spend two dollars for a hundred of these monstrosities instead of just going out and eating a carrot.

The same game goes on with ads for liver pills:

"Liver has been recognized by the nutritional and medical communities as one of the most important foods an individual can eat."

That's fine. Then they go on to tell you why their form of "desiccated" liver is the best, and how many vitamins and amino acids it contains. "Desiccated," by the way, is nothing more than a fancy word for "dried," but if you're selling plain old beef liver at three cents for 7½ grains you have to call it by some fancy name. The liver is chopped, then heated in a vacuum until it turns into a flaky powder. That's about the time it stopped being a "natural" product. In addition to other nutrients, all the vitamin C is murdered in the drying process. Oh, there's one other little detail. Beef liver costs about 89 cents a pound at the supermarket. Dried and powdered liver in capsules goes for $27.90 a pound, or about $27 a pound more than you should be paying. Besides, you pay a stranger to destroy some of the best vitamins in the product.

But what about organic vitamins?

Yes, what about organic vitamins? All vitamins are organic, some vitamins are organic, no vitamins are organic, and some vitamins are organic part of the time. All those statements are true—and anything else you want to say about organic and vitamins. The word *organic* is a copywriter's dream come true, since an unabridged dictionary lists at least fifteen separate definitions of *organic*. That makes anything and everything *organic* in some way or another.

Actually there is only one definition of *organic* that makes sense in relation to vitamins: *"Organic*—obtained directly from animal or vegetable sources." So vitamin C that is made by nature inside a tomato is organic vitamin C; vitamin C made in a chemist's test tube in the form of cevitamic acid is *not* organic vitamin C. Eat the tomato—that's why it exists. Leave the chemist to make more challenging things—like artificial-imitation-synthetic orange juice that glows in the dark.

Does the soil or climate where food is grown have anything to do with its vitamin or mineral content?

Of course it does. Just take one obvious example. Iodine is an essential mineral involved, among other things, in the regulation of the thyroid gland. Imagine that you performed an experiment by growing vegetables in soil that has no iodine. Do you think that the plant can manufacture iodine from thin air? Those vegetables will be totally lacking in iodine. People whose diet is composed of vegetables lacking in iodine may develop a disease called *goiter,* manifested by massive enlargement of the thyroid gland. For the past 200 years or so in the United States, exactly that sort of living experiment has been going on. In many parts of the Midwest, most of the iodine was drained from the soil by glaciers during the last Ice Age. Most of the vegetables grown in the affected area are deficient in iodine, so that the people who live there are extremely prone to develop iodine deficiencies. As a matter of fact, that entire section of the nation is known as the *goiter belt.*

The solution is obvious—the government could simply encourage farmers to add iodine to the soil with the rest of their fertilizer. Instead, they compel salt processors to add iodine to their salt—and mount expensive campaigns telling people to eat "iodized" salt.

Isn't that a good idea?

Not if you're sensitive to iodine—and some people are. They get skin rashes, allergies, and more serious problems from iodine, and most of the time they don't even know they're eating it. They make a special effort to buy uniodized salt, but restaurants, food processors, schools, and fast-food joints all dump large amounts of *iodized* salt into their products. It's really the same sort of nutritional bullying that goes on with so many other components of our daily diet. The "wise-fools" of the FDA tinker with our nutrition in a way that is convenient for the food processors—but not for us.

Why do you call them "wise-fools"?

Because that's what they are. The FDA and other similar government agencies that regulate food products (Department of Agriculture, Department of Commerce, etc.) have all the technical data about food at their fingertips. That's

51

the wise part. But the regulations they impose are the *apparently* foolish part.

For example, *FDA regulations make it a serious offense to make any of the following claims in relation to food:*

1. The presence of any substance in food has any relation to the cause or prevention of disease.
2. Transportation, storage, or cooking of food can reduce the nutrient content.
3. Food grown in inadequate soil may be deficient in nutrients.
4. Natural nutrients are better than imitation ones.

Any food product that makes those "claims" is considered "misbranded" and will be seized and destroyed with possible criminal action against the manufacturer and seller. But the FDA knows better than any of us that *all of the claims it prohibits are just and honest claims.*

For example?

Well, let's just take the example in the previous chapter. Deficiency of vitamin C in a diet can cause scurvy. A diet too low in vitamin B_1 causes beriberi. That's as obvious as it can be.

The second point is also well known. If you eat a raw pea, fresh from the pod in your backyard garden, you get 100 percent of the vitamins present in that pea. Take the pea right into your kitchen and cook it, and you cook away about 56 percent of the vitamins. That's unfortunate. But pay someone to pick, process and can that little pea for you, and this is what happens:

30 percent of the vitamins are lost in cooking at the canning plant
25 percent are lost in the process of sterilization
27 percent float away in the discarded liquid
12 percent are lost when you heat the canned pea after you open the can

You end up with a little round green disaster that has lost *94 percent* of the vitamins it started out with! Frozen peas are an improvement—they lose a mere *83 percent* of their vitamins in the course of being expensively processed for your dinner table. Like TV dinners? They lose up to *40 percent of their vitamin A, all of the vitamin C, 80 percent of all the B-complex vitamins,* and *over half of the vitamin E.* You could almost get more nutrition by sucking on the wrapper.

We've already mentioned the third point, the effect of inadequate soil on food. The U.S. Department of Agriculture, in its authoritative book, *Handbook Number 8,* points out, for example, that different varieties of oranges grown in different parts of the country have vitamin C contents ranging from 45 to 61 milligrams per unit measure. In addition, the amount of sunlight has a powerful effect on the vitamin content of a fruit or vegetable. Turnips, peaches, apples, and tomatoes that get *less sun contain less vitamins.* Storage of foods also depletes their nutrient content dramatically. For example, apples that are stored lose over half of their vitamin C content in the process.

Point four is a grim joke. The FDA has to insist that the cheap synthetic vitamins that are added to overprocessed refined flour, for example, are as good as the real honest-to-goodness vitamins placed there by Mother Nature. (Incidentally, when you think about it, Mother Nature is only another way of saying God, in these days when it is unfashionable to admit that there is any Higher Power than the computer.) Each and every one of the *scientists* who work for the FDA must turn their heads in shame when they hear their bosses proclaim that imitation nutrients are just as good as real foods.

Why does the FDA keep food sellers from telling the truth about food?

Because in food these days, the truth is too expensive. People pay hundreds of millions of dollars every year for junky *imitation* white bread. ("Imitation" is an accurate word because real bread is flour, water, yeast and salt. The white bread you see in the supermarket is quite a different product. See Chapter VIII.)

The purpose of Regulation 1 is to keep some sincere bread manufacturers from reminding the mommies and daddies of America that bad bread makes bad bodies.

Regulation 2 is necessary to keep the massive canning and freezing companies in business. The American people must not know that the vast majority of the vitamins in their food are efficiently removed when the product is canned, frozen, and otherwise preserved. How do you work that *news* into a TV commercial?

Regulation 3 keeps anyone from wondering about the hundreds of thousands of acres of fruit and vegetables that are grown in soil dangerously deficient in essential nutrients. Giant farming corporations add just enough nutrients to the soil to produce good-*looking* fruit and vegetables; they couldn't care less about the nutritional value, because it is against the law to tell consumers that one vital fact: food grown in deficient soil is deficient in nutrients. (If you don't believe it, scrape up some bad soil from a construction site and put it in a clay pot. Fill another pot with a good potting mix, and plant two identical house plants in the pots. Take identical care of them. In two weeks send the dead plant to the FDA.)

Regulation 4 is also necessary for the smooth flow of profits. Over 5000 chemical additives are poured into food products in America. The faintest suggestion that it's better to eat real food than imitation food can cause a drop in sales of the artificial product. The FDA doesn't want that.

Some people have gone so far as to suggest that these four FDA regulations violate the First (freedom of speech) Amendment of the U.S. Constitution. They provide police penalties for anyone who dares to tell the truth about food. It's an interesting theory.

Why do you think that the FDA is so slanted toward food processors?

I wasn't the first one to think of the possibility. For full details see Chapter XII.

CHAPTER IV
Minerals

Isn't it important to take plenty of iron?

No, it isn't. As a matter of fact, taking iron when you don't need it can lead to certain problems, including impotence and frigidity, heart failure, diabetes, and liver cancer.* But those nice young ladies who peddle iron tonics on television never tell you *that*.

Iron is a mineral, and unlike vitamins, you never use up your supply of iron. The average person has about 4 grams (or one seventh of an ounce) of the metal in his body; about two thirds of it is deposited in the red blood cells. Although red blood cells are scrapped about every four months, the iron is carefully recycled and used to make more red cells, so theoretically there is no need to take *any* iron into the body at all. Actually, however, there is a tiny daily loss of iron in feces, sweat, urine, and bile.

But don't women lose a lot of iron during their menstrual periods?

That's what the iron-tonic-and-snake-oil peddlers on TV would like you to believe. They say: "Because you're a

* *Merck Manual of Diagnosis and Treatment*, 12th ed. Rahway, N.J., Merck & Co., 1972, p. 1092.

woman, you have a very special need for iron. . . ." Kind of scary, isn't it? What they should really tell you is this:

"The average iron loss without menstruation is about half a milligram per day. During menstruation, the total loss of iron increases to an insignificant 1 milligram daily. The average woman in the U.S. and Europe consumes about 16 mg of iron daily, or sixteen times the maximum average loss during the menses."

But the trouble with the truth is it doesn't sell iron pills.

Aren't there some cases where people *should* take iron pills?

Of course. If you've just gotten rid of intestinal parasites called hookworms, if you've just had a serious blood loss, or if you're a baby whose mother feeds you on artificial formulas, you may need a small amount of extra iron.

The official Recommended Daily Allowance for iron is about 10 milligrams a day for adult men and 18 milligrams a day for adult women (sex discrimination!). It's about as far off as most of the other "official" recommendations. A woman who loses 1 mg per day total of iron during menstruation is supposed to take 240 mg a month extra to replace the 7 mg per month that she loses. That only makes sense if you're selling iron.

The iron recommendation for men, 10 mg daily, would seem to replace about $1/400$ of the body's stores daily but since only 5 percent of that is absorbed under normal conditions, an average man is replacing about $1/8000$ of his body total daily. That underlines the wisdom of depending on your daily diet to get your iron requirement.

But isn't it true that at least a quarter of all Americans suffer from iron-deficiency anemia?

That's what they said in the now discredited National Nutrition Survey—which cost the taxpayers a few million dollars, collapsed when the director quit in anger, and was never really completed.

If 50 million Americans actually suffered from iron-deficiency anemia, it would be a national emergency requiring drastic measures. It *is* true that the U.S. standard of living is declining (now third in the world after the Swiss and the Arabs), and it *is* true that the American diet becomes less nourishing every day, but those figures on anemia are false and misleading. They provide an excuse to merchandise iron pills, liquids, supplements, and other nostrums and distract public attention from the real problem—overprocessed and overchemicalized food.

What are the real facts about iron-deficiency anemia?

Here they are: Any mass survey of iron-deficiency anemia depends on a simple blood test that checks the amount of hemoglobin in the blood. Hemoglobin is a combination of iron and protein that helps carry oxygen from the lungs to all the tissues of the body; the four million or so red blood cells containing hemoglobin act like a tiny bucket brigade running back and forth twenty-four hours a day rushing oxygen wherever it is needed. *But a reduction in hemoglobin does not necessarily mean that the patient is suffering from iron-deficiency anemia.* Accurate diagnosis depends on expensive and complicated tests that are never done in mass surveys. (These include serum iron levels and sucking out bone marrow to measure iron.) Every doctor knows that most growing children develop an *apparent* anemia due to rapid growth and development. Pregnant women may also develop an *apparent* anemia due to an increase in the amount of liquid in the blood during pregnancy. (The same amount of iron diluted by more liquid gives a less-concentrated solution.) So an honest and responsible statement would be: "Fifty million Americans *appear* to be suffering from iron-deficiency anemia. Of these, approximately 49 million either do not have anemia or will restore their iron stores from their diet without incident."

Can a person cure himself of iron-deficiency anemia?

Yes. Once the basic cause is treated by the doctor (such as bleeding ulcer, intestinal parasites, extra-heavy menstruation, or the like), the body has startling ways to heal itself. In the case of iron deficiency, the body automatically increases iron absorption 400 percent until the anemia is cured. Then it cuts iron absorption to the old level of about 5 percent of iron intake. As the medical texts put it:

"In adults, unless the diet is grossly abnormal, deficient iron intake is generally an inadequate explanation for hypochromic (iron-deficiency) anemia."*

But it's not too hard to give your baby anemia.

How does that happen?

Most of the popular and widely sold baby formulas—basically mixtures of cheap powdered skim milk, refined sugar, and coconut oil—contain no more than a "trace" (whatever *that* is) of iron. An infant requires, from birth to two months, about *6 milligrams of iron daily;* from two months to six months, about *10 milligrams of iron daily.* A baby who gets nothing more than the iron-deficient widely advertised "formulas" starts off life with a guaranteed iron-deficiency anemia; his challenge is to survive for the first few months of life with only the iron he was born with.

But can't the mother give the baby iron drops?

Sure. The same companies that sell the iron-deficient imitation milks sell iron drops. They only cost a couple of dollars a bottle, can cause fatal iron poisoning in excess dosage, and provide iron in a form that is difficult to absorb. Alternatively, a mother can breast-feed her baby and

* *AMA Drug Evaluations,* 1st ed., American Medical Association, Chicago, 1971.

provide about 1 milligram of *organic* iron per quart of human milk—free.*

Babies fed on drugstore formulas are virtually the only example of iron-deficiency anemia due to diet in modern countries. Ironically "modern" mothers pay hundreds of millions of dollars a year to make their babies anemic. Where are we going?

For babies fed on cow's milk (worse than human milk but better than the skim-milk-sugar-and-coconut-oil commercial formulas), a good source of iron is a little freshly squeezed orange juice daily or, later on, some egg yolk—both containing about 1 milligram of iron per ounce.

How can adults be sure of getting enough iron?

It's easy. All they have to do is eat like intelligent adults —instead of pawns of the food and vitamin pill industries. The average American diet contains about 16 milligrams of iron a day. That's not as good as it used to be—the ignorant (and underprivileged?) English peasants back in 1400 were consuming about 21 mg of iron daily. But if you want to forget about the whole problem, just make sure your food is cooked in old-fashioned (unenameled) iron pots and pans. That alone can give you about 20 mg of iron free—more if you cook acid foods like spaghetti sauce and other tomato-based dishes.† Other good sources of dietary iron are meat, whole wheat products, and wheat bran, which contains about 5 mg of iron per ounce.

What about foods that are supplemented with iron?

Yes, that's a new wrinkle, isn't it? Most breakfast cereals, especially those for kids, have a big shot of iron added. Some of the best-selling brands have as much as 25 mg of iron per ounce. That much iron costs a fraction of a penny,

* Jackson et al.: Growth of well-born American infants fed human and cow's milk. *Pediatrics,* 33:642, 1964.

† Goodhart, R. S.: *Modern Nutrition in Health and Disease,* 5th ed. Philadelphia, Lea & Febiger, 1973.

looks good on the label, and supplies in one ounce twice as much iron as the average 11- to 14-year-old needs all day. Not only is that an insult to the intelligence of the parents, but it can be downright dangerous.

How can taking too much iron be dangerous?

Excessive iron builds *bad* bodies in two ways. First, recent studies have shown that humans with a high iron intake encourage the growth of dangerous bacteria within their bodies, including the potentially fatal *E. coli.**
That may be one of the reasons why the incidence of serious infections which *do not respond to antibiotics* has been increasing. Animals have a very low concentration of iron in their blood and prevent bacteria from multiplying by literally starving them into extinction. Nature sees to everything: human milk has its iron locked up in a special iron-protein complex which makes it available to baby and unavailable to bacteria.

What's the other danger from taking too much iron?

A terrible disease known as *hemochromatosis.* Those heartrending iron tonic commercials on TV should occasionally show a victim of this incurable malady. Massive iron deposits build up in vital organs of the body and produce sexual impotence, diabetes, heart failure, and ultimately liver cancer. The pitiful victims also end up with their skin permanently stained a peculiar bronze color—looking like they got a strange suntan from outer space. There is no cure but there is a treatment: you go to the doctor and once a week he drains half a quart of blood from your veins and pours it down the sink. A high alcohol intake hastens the iron deposits, and ironically most of the liquid iron "tonics" are up to 30-proof drinking alcohol—to give the consumer an instant "high."
So taking iron supplements can be a nuisance, expose

---

* Dr. Ivan Kochan, University of Miami, Oxford, Ohio, reported to the American Chemical Society convention, 1976.

you to infection, mar your appearance (by staining your teeth), poison your little kids if they get into the fruit-flavored iron liquid in the medicine chest, and perhaps give you a rare and incurable disease. It's also expensive. If you buy 150-mg tabs—far more than you need—for 2 cents each, you are paying a whopping $64 a pound for the *equivalent* of iron rust. It hardly seems worth it.

What about phytic acid? I've heard that it interferes with the absorption of iron.

That's right. But another way to say it might be: "Phytic acid limits the absorption of iron to prevent serious damage from excessive iron intake." And that's the way it really is.

Phytic acid is a very interesting story. When the high-fiber diet first became popular, food processors were caught with their fiber (content) down. They desperately needed something to frighten their customers—that means you—away from fiber until they could unload their low-fiber junk foods. After a desperate search, some of their consultants—who were professors of nutrition and should have known better—came up with the "demon" of phytic acid. They shrieked that phytic acid "prevented the absorption of essential minerals such as iron and zinc" and had actually produced deficiencies in "susceptible populations." The campaign gathered steam as an entire section of the national convention of a well-known scientific organization was devoted to attacking the idea of the high-fiber diet and suggesting idiocies such as "fiber can scratch your stomach" or "fiber will give you cancer of the liver."

Is any of that true?

Of course not. What is true is that the white sugar, white bread, pasta, and pastry that Americans eat have given them more chronic disease than any other nation in the world. Now let's take a look at what "phytic acid" really is.

Its real name is "inositolhexaphosphoric acid," and it is

found in whole wheat and some other whole grains. The *only* cases of mineral deficiencies due to phytic acid that have ever been found were in a group of Iranian peasants who subsisted almost exclusively on *unleavened* whole wheat bread. That's 100 percent whole wheat bread made without yeast or baking power, and you couldn't get one American in a million to touch it. Most of the phytic acid is destroyed by the leavening in the baking process (yeast or baking powder), and you can thank God—literally—for what remains.

What do you mean, "Thank God—literally"?

Just that. The food companies with their wonderful full-page ads would like you to believe that your food as God made it is some kind of terrible mistake. Like phytic acid in your bread will make you into some kind of circus dwarf unless Pan-International-United Bakers, Inc., comes to your rescue with their bright-white-cottonlike-melt-in-your-mouth-imitation-bread. That's not the way it is. Phytic acid is part of the Master Plan for the human race, and it stands between you and excess absorption of dangerous minerals.

As the consumption of whole grains—*with their phytic acid content*—has gone *down,* the incidence of kidney stones *from excess mineral absorption* has gone up. More than that, among people who don't get enough phytic acid (that is, Americans and western Europeans) there is a veritable epidemic of calcium kidney stones—the kind that are excruciatingly painful and can cause permanent disability and death. That phytic acid that the food processors want to "protect" you from traps the excess calcium and prevents it from being absorbed by your body. You still get all the calcium you need but not in your kidneys where it can kill you.*

So instead of all those complaints, let's hear a cheer for phytic acid, the first line of defense against kidney stones!

---

* Gibbon, N.: Urological implications of food refining. *European Urology,* 1:36–37, 1975.

So what should a person do about getting the right amount of iron?

Next to nothing. Cook your food in iron pots, eat fresh fruits and vegetables, whole wheat bread, and whole grain cereals, and keep as far as you can from any food product that has iron artificially added to it. Don't—under any circumstances—pop iron pills unless your doctor specifically recommends it. Those pills are potentially dangerous and can cause fatal and incurable diseases. They can also k"l your little kids if they find the bottle and swallow a few mouthfuls. Remember that 99 percent of tiredness is emotional, and under those circumstances even 500 tons of iron would only give you a heavy feeling. The people who peddle iron tonics know all that—but they care about profits, not about your health. That says it clearly, I think.

Since I started reading this book I've been looking at the labels on vitamin bottles and food packages, and I see that vitamin and mineral contents of foods and pills are expressed in "MDR" and "RDA." Where do those terms come from?

Outer space. The most commonly used term, RDA, stands for "Recommended Dietary Allowance." MDR stands for "Minimum Daily Requirement" and is about as worthless.

Until recently the Food and Drug Administration had its own set of vitamin and mineral recommendations called "Minimum Daily Requirements." In reality these were nothing more than touched-up copies of the RDAs. But then, the FDA decided to call its recommendations by 'he same name. So we have government RDAs and non-governmental RDAs. When the poor consumer sees "RDA" on a label, he can't be sure where it comes from. But he *can* be sure of one thing.

What's that?

That the Recommended Dietary Allowances recommend much more than he really needs. Just by chance, there's another organization that calculates vitamin and mineral needs—this time from a medical and official government point of view. It's called the Food and Agricultural Organization of the World Health Organization. If we compare their findings with those of the giant food companies, we find some very interesting things:

The following figures compare the World Health Organization recommendations with the FDA and "Food and Nutrition Board" recommendations for an adult man:*

Vitamin A: FDA suggests 100% *more.*
Vitamin B₁: FDA recommends 125% *more.*
Niacin: FDA recommends 133% *more.*
Folic acid: FDA recommends 250% *more.*
B₁₂: FDA recommends 250% *more.*
Vitamin C: FDA recommends 200% *more.*
Calcium: FDA recommends 200% *more.*
Iron: FDA recommends 143% *more.*

So we have the strange situation of the Food and Drug Administration of the United States recommending from 100 to 250 percent more vitamins and minerals than all the learned medical experts in the entire rest of the world combined. But the funny thing is that *the United States has the shortest life expectancy of any comparable country.*

---

* Taken from Scrimshaw and Young: Requirements for human nutrition. *Scientific American,* Sept. 1976.

I've read a lot about milk as a source of calcium and phosphorus. What do you think of that?

Sheer extravagance, that's what I think. Let's look at what calcium is all about and you'll see why I feel that way. The average adult body contains about 2¾ pounds of calcium, most of it in the bones and teeth. But calcium is a two-edged sword. As we've seen, if you consume too much of it, it can accumulate in your kidneys, form kidney stones, and ruin your life. So the body has a series of complicated and delicate mechanisms to keep too much calcium from getting into your blood. Phytic acid in your diet helps, and the body rejects about 80 percent of all the calcium you eat to keep your blood concentration relatively low. If the amount in your blood gets too low, the parathyroid gland produces a hormone which releases some of the calcium from your bones so you can use it. But if you meddle too much with your diet, your body can get swamped with calcium and then it piles up in the kidneys. The dairy industry in the United States wants to sell massive amounts of cow's milk because there's big money in milk. (If you doubt that, ask yourself why, in these days of inflation, milk is the only basic food which has *reverse price control*. Authorities *set a minimum price for milk and it cannot be legally sold for less*.)

Anyhow, the dairy people want you to think that you should drink milk—that's why they had that cute little million-dollar advertising campaign telling you: "Every Body Needs Milk!" The Federal Trade Commission objected and finally the campaign was dropped but the message got through. Everybody *doesn't* need milk, and more than half the people in the world—including nearly a quarter of the people in the United States—can get sick if they drink milk. (Full details on that later.)

The World Health Organization says you need 500 milligrams of calcium a day. The FDA, with a push from the dairy associations, says you need 1200 milligrams a day. That overdose will cost you 45 cents a day for each member of your family, if you're foolish enough to try to get it from milk. Milk is also perishable, needs refrigeration, and can make you fat.

Alternatively you can pick up a bunch of turnip greens from the corner grocery—free if you buy the turnips. They will help you lose weight, won't spoil at room temperature, and *weight-for-weight contain twice as much calcium as milk!* You never saw *that* on a billboard, did you? Those turnip greens will also give you plenty of phosphorus free in the bargain.

You don't like turnip greens? Try whole wheat bread. It contains half as much calcium by weight as milk plus a bit of phytic acid to protect you even more. Or try beans, olives, peanuts—dozens of other vegetables which have more calcium than you can use. And remember, there is virtually no possibility of a calcium deficiency in a normal person. You get plenty in your diet and the body stores it well, so you don't have to eat it every day.

If you don't need extra calcium, why do they sell calcium pills?

For the same reason they sell mink coats—to make money. If you're tired of working for a living and are looking for a nice business, consider selling calcium in pill form. This is how to go about it:

First compose your ads—there are plenty around to copy from. They say things like: "Get your vital life-giving calcium from deep within snow-capped mountains in the form of fresh sparkling dolomite!"

Sound good? Then price your pills attractively—say, 2 cents each for a 44-grain dolomite tablet. Then stand back and watch the orders pour in. What's dolomite? Oh, yes.

Dolomite is a white mineral composed of calcium carbonate (otherwise known as chalk) and magnesium carbonate. That white rock they use on the roofs in your neighborhood may well be dolomite. Of course, you'll have to pay $4 to have a ton of it delivered to your garage or wherever you make your pills. That comes out to a whopping penny for 5 pounds. But don't worry, you'll be collecting $16 for that same 5 pounds. Let's see, that's about a 160,000 percent markup. Of course, there will be expenses, but even if they are 1000 percent of sales, that still leaves you with 159,000 percent profit. Not bad.

What about phosphorus?

Phosphorus plays second fiddle to calcium in bone and tooth metabolism, and it's almost impossible to develop a deficiency unless you have some terrible disease. The whole question of vitamins and minerals is much like the mechanics of breathing. If you start to think about how many times a minute and how deeply you should breathe—and try to control it—you'll get into big trouble. The best solution to getting your vitamins and minerals is just to eat a natural diet consisting of fresh, wholesome, unprocessed foods as God intended you to.

How come you talk so much about God? What is this, a nutrition book or a religious tract?

Maybe you'd call it a "nutritional tract." Look at it this way. A plain old apple contains 191 known chemical compounds, each of which plays an important role in human nutrition. When you eat that apple, over 1300 chemical reactions occur to break it down into its component molecules. Those molecules are then dispatched to exactly the areas of the body where they are required. The pectin goes to the large intestine, the vitamin C is sent to the skin, the vitamin A goes to the retinal area of the eyes, and so on times 191. *You* don't make it happen because you don't even *know* it's happening. There are 160,000 edible plants on this earth—you didn't put any of them there. But most of them help keep you alive. Your digestive system was designed by God—not by you and not by IBM and not by a government agency. It can take almost any animal that walks by or any plant that springs up in an empty field and convert it into brain, bone, heart, and muscle to keep you alive. Even the most arrogant and self-important "scientist" must admit that a Being far wiser than any human must have devised and implemented that still-uncomprehended nutritional system.

So don't think that the people who make instant breakfasts or imitation orange juice or yucky white imitation bread have the slightest idea what your body needs. That applies as well to those who turn out vitamin pills and nutritional supplements. Those fumbling human brains cannot improve on the Master Design that brought you here and allows you to survive from day to day.

CHAPTER V
Trace Elements

I've heard that it's important to get enough salt. Is that true?

It certainly is. But the real challenge in most "modern" countries is to keep yourself from being pickled by the salt in your daily diet. Salt is composed of two vital chemical elements: sodium and chlorine. Its chemical name is sodium chloride. It is present in every body fluid, including blood, sperm, spinal fluid, digestive juices, and is found within every cell. But the amount of salt you need to stay healthy is very very small. For the average man it amounts to 200 milligrams a day, or about one twentieth of a teaspoonful. The average American who gorges on processed food consumes about 20 grams, or almost a full ounce of salt a day! That's about 100 times what his body needs and adds up to big trouble.

Why does it add up to trouble?

It's the sodium that causes the damage. One of the few things that almost all doctors agree on is that a high intake of sodium is a vital factor in causing high blood pressure. (The medical name for high blood pressure is *hypertension*. That doesn't mean that you are "tense"—it means that the blood flows through your arteries with much too much pressure, damaging your blood vessels, your heart,

71

and your brain.) High blood pressure causes over 150,000 deaths a year in the United States alone—that's about 17 dead people every hour. High salt consumption is not the only cause of high blood pressure, but it is a very important contributing factor, especially in three vital areas.

What areas are those?

First, a high salt intake in infancy and childhood predisposes to later high blood pressure. Second, people who are on the brink of high blood pressure can often avoid it by restricting their consumption of salt. Third, those who already have hypertension can often avoid the complications, such as heart attack, stroke, blindness, and paralysis, by drastically cutting down on their salt intake.

But for most people it's a much more difficult task than it may seem.

Why is that?

Well, most natural *unprocessed* food is relatively low in sodium. But most processed and factory-made food is overdosed with sodium in the form of salt and other additives. There is an obvious reason for that: the mechanics of processing food generally leave it flat and tasteless. A big slug of salt literally poisons your taste buds and makes overcooked, overprocessed food semipalatable. A good example is the tasty little pea.

If you bring the fresh peas in from the garden and pop them into the pot, they will contain about 1 milligram of sodium per 100 grams (about 3 ounces). Warm up the same amount of canned peas and you'll sock yourself with about *240* milligrams of sodium in the form of salt. That's a mere 239,000 percent increase in potentially deadly sodium—necessary to make a pale mushy canned pea barely swallowable. Frozen peas fare better; they only suffer a 128,000 percent increase in salt to cover up the flat frozen taste. The canning industry generally adds more than half of 1 percent by weight of salt to canned vegetables—enough to do you plenty of harm if you have a tendency to high blood pressure. Just to prove they can do it, they also make a low-sodium product for those who have had too much salt already. Typically those contain 3 milligrams of sodium per 3 ounces—and taste awful, as any overcooked vegetable does.

Are all processed foods loaded with salt?

Let's look at a few examples:

Dried soups from envelopes: 1000 mg of sodium per serving
Cheese spreads: 1600 mg of sodium per serving
Boxed cookies: 500 mg of sodium per serving
Margarine: 1000 mg of sodium per serving
Breakfast cereal: average, 1200 to 1400 mg of sodium per serving
Italian-style salad dressing: 2000 mg of sodium per serving
Bran flakes: 1000 mg of sodium per serving
Natural bran: a mere 9 mg of sodium per serving
Typical frozen "TV" dinner: 2000 mg of sodium per serving

Once you venture into the fast-food jungle along the side of the highway, you are lost. Hamburgers, hot dogs, chicken, pizza, fish-and-chips, french-fried potatoes, sandwiches, and all the rest of the offerings are so loaded with salt that the companies involved will not reveal the actual sodium content. But that's not the worst of the pickling of America.

What's the worst?

It's really a conspiracy against the children of America, using mothers as the unwilling "hit-women."

First, let's look at what might be called "the dog-food caper." Dogs, you see, have very special tastes in food. The flavor experts who work for the biggest food companies have spent hundreds of thousands of dollars discovering that your family pooch prefers a meal that tastes like a dead fish that has been in the sun for about a week. The ideal flavor, to quote from a technical food industry article on the subject, is as follows:

"The predominant note should be decaying fish flesh with rancid and putrid overtones. When offered these samples, test dogs not only ate voraciously but overturned the plates and rolled in the product."

Of course, dog *owners* don't like the smell of rotten fish around the house, so the food has to be gussied up for them. It is dyed a nice pink, or made to look like hamburger, or molded like imitation chops—and ultimately so transformed that it is a wonder more dog owners don't fight their pups for a plateful of "Super Bow-Wow Cutlets."

Well, that's the way it is with commercial baby food. Milk, baby's first food, is a bland food, low in salt and sodium. Babies will eat bland low-sodium baby foods eagerly, precisely because they taste so much like milk. But Mommy won't. Mother always tastes the baby food, and it has to taste at least passably good to *her*. But her taste buds have been packed in salt for so many years that she wrinkles up her nose at any baby food that doesn't have at least the same slug of salt as the canned peas she innocently inflicts on the family. So baby-food manufacturers usually add the same amount of salt to baby foods as they do to the adult products. That's fine for Mom, with her big well-developed kidneys that *might* be able to dispose of that massive dose of sodium. But baby kidneys are tiny little things no bigger than a grape, and they just can't deal with all that salt. Many specialists in hypertension believe that one of the worst causes of the disease is massive amounts of salt in infancy. On the other hand, it sells baby food. Then baby-food makers went one step farther—and almost literally made us a nation of idiots.

What did they do?

They used another chemical to dope up the baby's dinner so Mom would like her occasional spoonful even better. You know that very special taste Chinese restaurant food has? The taste you can really never get at home? That's because the Chinese add a chemical derived from soybeans or sugar beets called *monosodium glutamate* (MSG for short). The real magic of MSG is that it can make a tired flabby canned vegetable or meat product taste *almost* fresh again. So MSG was pumped into baby food. Then one of those funny little coincidences happened. A Chinese doctor living in the United States noticed that whenever he went out to eat in a Chinese restaurant, he came home feeling dizzy, light-headed and generally weird. He finally traced it to the MSG used in the restaurant food, and with a rare sense of humor christened his condition "CRS" or "Chinese Restaurant Syndrome." It then developed that a lot of other doctors and just plain people suffered from the same symptoms, but no one had connected it with MSG. That sparked some animal experiments which proved once and for all that MSG can cause *severe irreversible brain damage* in baby mice, rats, chicks, and monkeys. There's no reason to wait around and see if it will do the same to infant humans.

The Food and Drug Administration examined the evidence and decided that, for all they cared, American babies could eat MSG until they grew up and became directors of the FDA. But the controversy got into the newspapers, the mothers of America were aroused, and the baby-food manufacturers beat a hasty retreat. As they were falling all over themselves to take the MSG out of the baby jars, they issued a mountain of press releases telling us how great the product was. That didn't surprise anyone. So all your babies have to contend with now is little jars full of awful starch, refined sugar, and massive amounts of salt.

But don't you have to eat plenty of salt to get enough iodine?

No. There was a period in the history of the world when people had a lot of confidence in SCIENCE. That's when they believed "scientists" would ultimately solve all the world's most pressing problems. Remember? Men in white coats were going to reduce all our nutritional needs to one little pill we could take three times a day. Instead they gave us the atomic bomb, napalm, and nerve gas. But in the process, when we still had all that confidence in them, they decided we needed more iodine in our diet. There was some basis in those days for feeling that way. Many thousands of years ago gigantic rivers of ice, glaciers, raked their way across what was to become the United States. As the glaciers receded they pulled some of the minerals out of the soil, including a lot of iodine in the area between the Rocky Mountains and the Appalachians and from the Canadian border south. Since there was almost no iodine in the soil in these areas, there was hardly any iodine in the fruits and vegetables grown there.* That resulted in chronic thyroid deficiency in some, but not all, of the people in those areas. The "scientists" decided they had to force these folks to eat iodine, and they looked for some way to compel them to consume the chemical. Finally they decided to add iodine to salt, reasoning correctly that everyone had to eat salt and so there was no way they could avoid getting iodine. Fortunately at the last minute, they remembered that some people are poisoned by small amounts of iodine. So they allowed the manufacture of *uniodized* salt as well. (Incidentally they did a more thorough job with the fluoride question. If you live where they put fluoride in your water—without your consent— you get fluoride, without your consent.)

The amount usually added to salt is about .01 percent potassium iodine, which *may not* do you any harm, but which also doesn't really belong in your salt shaker either.

---

* That scientific finding, incidentally, contradicts the FDA regulation that insists that the soil has no effect on the vitamin or mineral content of food that is grown in it. Hmmmm.

If it's harmless why shouldn't it be in your salt shaker?

For three very good reasons. First, adding iodine to your salt opened the door to dosing salt with a whole bunch of chemicals that really have no place in your diet. For example, some salt manufacturers have taken to adding up to 2 percent silicon dioxide to your salt to keep it from caking. I don't like that in my salt and you won't like it in your salt when I tell you what it is. It's *sand*. It's also good business; salt is cheap but sand is cheaper. They save 2 percent on the cost of the product—without lowering the price—by letting you swallow sand. Sand is also heavier than salt, and since salt is sold by weight . . . well, you can figure it out. You may also find any of the following in your salt: aluminum calcium silicate, magnesium silicate, calcium silicate, sodium aluminosilicate, sodium calcium aluminosilicate, or tricalcium silicate—all variations on that theme. Other salt sellers dope up their product with yellow prussiate of soda or sodium ferrocyanide. That doesn't belong on your soft-boiled eggs either.

Second, there are some people who are allergic or sensitive to iodine. They try to avoid iodized salt when they can, but restaurant, military, college, and factory cafeteria food can be loaded with it. They get dosed with iodine against their will.

Third—and most important—it is no longer necessary to add iodine to salt; in fact iodized salt may just be the thing that gives you a harmful overdose of iodine.

How can just a little iodine in salt give an overdose?

Like this:

Things have changed since the 1920s; with efficient food distribution in the United States, people consume fruits and vegetables from outside the iodine-deficient areas of the country. So they get plenty of iodine from that part of their diet. In addition there is plenty of iodine in dairy products and seafood, which people eat more of lately.

But the key to the whole problem is factory-made bread.

These days, bread is made in gigantic mixes like so much cement. To make the dough easier to manage, the manufacturers (please don't call them "bakers" anymore) add chemicals to "condition" the dough and give it a plastic consistency. The "conditioner" is most likely to be *potassium iodate* in amounts up to 75 parts per million. That means a single slice of bread can have a whopping 2 milligrams of iodine! That adds up to 100 percent more than the desirable intake for a whole day. Six slices of bread a day plus iodized salt plus the iodine in an average modern diet can sock you with close to 1000 percent of your iodine requirement every day. There is a condition known as "iodine-excess goiter," which is massive enlargement of the thyroid gland caused by too much iodine.

So that's three reasons why iodine doesn't belong in your salt—and the goiter it may cause is just as bad as the goiter that comes from too little iodine.

What about some of the other minerals?

Well, let's take a fast trip through the most important minerals in alphabetical order, starting with aluminum. You won't see any aluminum pills in the drugstore because aluminum is a deadly poison. I've always wondered about the safety of aluminum pots and pans, since it has been established over and over again that some aluminum is absorbed into food cooked in aluminum vessels. Ancient Rome was supposed to have declined because the wealthiest and most capable citizens ate and drank from expensive lead utensils, producing chronic lead poisoning. I know that manufacturers of aluminum pots insist that there are no ill effects from the aluminum you absorb from their products. The symptoms of chronic aluminum poisoning are constipation, loss of appetite, and loss of energy.

Cadmium is another hazardous metal, although recently it has become fashionable to call metals found in your diet "trace elements." It may sound more impressive and the word "trace" may imply it can't be hazardous, but to chemists cadmium is just plain old cadmium.

Cadmium is very poisonous and may play a role in increasing the already astronomical incidence of heart attacks. (In the United States these days, over 2000 people every day *die* of heart attacks.) Most of the cadmium gets into your food courtesy of the food processors. It can be found in refined sugar and polished white rice, thanks to the refining procedures. The plumbing in your house can also zap you with plenty of cadmium, since water softeners, galvanized pipes, and black plastic pipes can all release the metal into your drinking water. No one should swallow even a milligram of deadly cadmium if he can help it.

Chromium is an important metal which is necessary in very small amounts. Unfortunately the same refining process that puts cadmium into your diet takes the chromium out.

What's the solution?

One solution is to eat grains. You avoid most of the dangerous metals, get the desirable ones, and also get the protection of phytic acid in the process—all free! Most of the necessary metals and minerals are present in the wheat germ and the wheat bran—discarded in the refining process.

Just one example illustrates the point. Every year *thirty-two billion* milligrams of vitamin B₆ are poured into the sewers of America in the process of converting nutritious whole wheat flour into nearly worthless white flour. If we consider the value as only 2 cents for two milligrams of B₆ at retail, that adds up to $320 million wasted in just *one* unnecessary refining process.

Cobalt is another "trace element" of obscure function. Vitamin B₁₂ contains cobalt, but nobody really knows what role the metal plays in the economy of the body.

Copper is another interesting substance in human nutrition. Everyone agrees that copper is too poisonous to be used in pots and pans. Those utensils that are made of copper have a protective layer of tin between the food and the copper bottom. Yet many multivitamin tablets sold at the drugstore or by mail contain as much as one milligram of copper. That brings to mind two interesting questions:

1. If copper is too dangerous to cook in but safe enough to swallow in pills, and aluminum is too dangerous to put into pills, how come aluminum is safe to cook in?
2. Since there has never been a case of copper deficiency in the history of the world, why are people being sold copper in pills at $9600 a pound (assuming a retail price of 2 cents a pill) when they can buy purer copper for about 75 cents a pound?

But that's nothing compared to the problem with fluoride.

What's the problem with fluoride?

The fluoride that is added to drinking water and toothpaste in the United States these days is probably one of the best examples of ignorance triumphing over science. Or maybe it's greed triumphing over ignorance. Whatever you want to call it, it's pretty scary.

The traditional lineup in the so-called fluoride controversy has been the political ultraconservatives on one side complaining about government interference with their water supply, and the so-called enlightened and progressive parts of the community supporting a measure to improve the public health. But there's an easy way to decide whether that chemical, sodium fluoride, belongs in the drinking water you give your kids.

What's the easy way?

Just take a cool analytical look at what fluoride is and the effect it has on human beings. The reasoning behind adding fluoride to your drinking water is based on the discovery that areas of the world which have a relatively *high* level of naturally occurring fluoride in the water have a relatively *low* level of tooth decay. Therefore, according to the public health "experts," the best way to decrease tooth decay is to artificially add fluorides to the water. That's actually about the worst way to cut down on tooth decay. First of all, it follows the current pattern of "modern medicine" in that it ignores the cause of a disease. Tooth decay is *not* produced by a deficiency of fluorides. It is produced by eating refined carbohydrates like white flour, white sugar, refined cereals, and all the other refined junk that make up the most profitable food products sold to unsuspecting consumers, many of them little kids. Instead of taking that terrible sugar glaze off the children's cereal, instead of cutting down on the refined sugar in food products that don't need sugar, it's better business to sell yet another grossly overpriced product—a fluoridating plant plus chemicals—to every big city and small town in the nation. Tooth decay produced by the products sold also opens up a new and sensationally profitable market for toothpaste doped up with fluoride.

Those fluoride plants are especially nice, since politicians buy them with other people's money—yours and mine—and they don't really worry about how much they cost. But there's something about those fluoride plants that's not so nice. They set the precedent of adding a controversial chemical to the water. If the "experts" decide today that we should have fluorides in our tea, coffee, frozen orange juice, lemonade, *and every cell of our bodies,* what's in store for us tomorrow? What about vitamin C in the water, considered by some to be much more important than fluoride? What about tranquilizers to avoid civil disorders? What about birth-control chemicals to be routed to the water in certain ethnic neighborhoods? When the time comes, of course, you can be sure it will be done for "your comfort and safety."

But is fluoride *that* bad?

You be the judge. Sodium *fluoride,* the chemical added to drinking water, is a deadly poison, a thousand times more deadly than the sodium *chloride*, or table salt, with which it is deceptively compared. (Generally speaking, adding fluoride to a formula makes a substance explosively active. Hydro*chloric* acid will eat through *copper;* hydro*fluoric* acid can't be kept in bottles because it eats through *glass!*) Just a little too much sodium fluoride causes convulsions, coma, and death. The maximum safe dose of fluoride, according to the United States Public Health Service,* is about *one milligram* per day. (Remember that one milligram is one thousandth of a gram, and one gram is about one thirtieth of an ounce. It isn't a whole lot of anything.) The average person gets about 0.45 mg of fluoride from his diet, about 1 mg from his fluoridated toothpaste (if he "brushes after every meal"), and up to 1.6 mg a day from fluoridated water. That adds up to a total intake of 3.05 mg a day of fluoride. Everyone agrees that intakes of about 2 mg a day can very likely cause permanent spotting of the teeth. Those big black blotches especially prominent on the front teeth don't look too good on your 14-year-old daughter who is just getting interested in boys. It's better for her to just cut down on her refined sugar and refined flour intake. But that's nothing compared to the other problem with excess fluoride.

It has been conclusively proved that women who take in more than 2 mg of fluorine per day *have a much greater chance of giving birth to mentally defective children*. Maybe those blackened teeth are nature's way of keeping girls who get a lot of fluorine from ever getting to that stage. If it sounds terrible, it *is* terrible.

But aren't the risks of taking fluoride justified by the protection it gives?

Hardly. Fluoride doesn't really protect against tooth decay. It merely *partially* undoes the damage caused by eating refined sugar and refined flour. Instead of exposing your entire body—and that includes your genes and chromo-

* Prinz et al., *Pharmacology & Dental Therapeutics*, 9th ed. St. Louis, C. V. Mosby.

somes—to a powerful and toxic chemical, just stop eating junk that rots your teeth. Too simple?

What about lead?

Well, Americans will never have to worry about a lead deficiency. They get tons of lead absolutely free. The only trouble is, lead is a deadly poison and is found nowadays in almost everything you breathe, eat, or drink. You will find it in smoke from your favorite brand of cigarette—there may be low-tar and -nicotine brands, but so far there's no "low-lead" cigarette, although lead is far deadlier than tar and nicotine combined. Lead is in your drinking water from pipes or from contaminated rivers and lakes. Lead is in cosmetics and the glazes on dinner plates. Lead is in the paints on walls and ceilings. Lead pours into your lungs straight from the exhaust pipes of *130 million* motor vehicles in the United States. You can even get your daily deadly dose of lead from the dinner table. Fruits and vegetables grown near heavily traveled highways collect significant amounts of lead. Cows and sheep that graze in pastures bathed in automobile exhaust concentrate lead in their meat and organs.

Lead is really a deadly poison—there's no doubt about that. The poisonous dose is about one milligram—that means two pounds of food with as little as one part per million of lead contamination can cause lead poisoning. The major symptoms of lead poisoning are anemia, weakness, headache, and fatigue. Higher doses may cause degeneration of the brain, which may explain one of the problems of the politicians who let so much lead get into our environment in the first place.

Isn't it unkind to say that?

You be the judge. The major cause of lead poisoning in the United States is the lead in gasoline. It gets there in the form of a substance called *tetraethyl lead*—that's what you're asking for when you say, "Fill 'er up with ethyl!" There is some lead in so-called regular gasoline too. The lead is put into the gasoline because it cuts down on knocking, allowing cars to have big, powerful, high-performance engines. Cars can run just as well, actually better, on gasoline that has very little lead, so-called low-lead gas. So your favorite politicians passed a law making gas stations sell low-lead gas and forcing the car manufacturers to choke off the filler pipe of your new car so you can't easily get the high-lead gas into your tank. That infuriated a lot of motorists and increased the sale of funnels. The whole process was dumb basically because they sell "low-lead" gas for a few cents *more* than high-lead gas. If *you* were doing it, you'd sell the low-lead gas for two cents a gallon *less* than the high-lead type, and that's what most of us would buy. And most of the lead would go out of the atmosphere within a week or so. (Politicians look down on that kind of solution and call it "simplistic." That means it's simple and saves taxpayers money.) In this case, it would also save lives.

What are some of the other important minerals?

Mercury is an especially lethal poison that has probably gotten into your stomach a couple of times already since you got out of bed this morning. But the mercury problem is so serious that it deserves special treatment in a later chapter.

Selenium is another deadly "trace element" that should never be added to your diet. It is useful in the treatment of a disease called *kwashiorkor*, which you are unlikely to ever hear of again now that you have seen it in print. There has never been a case in the United States, Canada, or Europe.

Magnesium is a relatively nontoxic metal that *is* essential. You don't have to worry about getting enough of it, since it is a component of chlorophyll and found in all green vegetables plus whole grains. You can also get it in those famous dolomite pills if you like to lick rocks. Your body is superb at handling magnesium—along with every other nutrient. When your magnesium stores are low, you will absorb three quarters of all the magnesium you swallow. When you have enough magnesium for the moment, three quarters of the magnesium you eat is excreted. No healthy person in the history of the world has ever had a magnesium deficiency—but that doesn't mean you can't buy magnesium pills! At one cent each for 50 milligrams they will run you over $90 a pound for magnesium carbonate. The retail price of that common chemical should be about 80 cents a pound—at most. Not a bad profit on something you don't need. Enjoy!

Another interesting metal is nickel. It's a good example of the problems of peddling refined foods. You don't have to worry about a lack of nickel—the danger is slow cumulative metal poisoning as in the case of cadmium, aluminum, and lead. Nickel doesn't belong in your diet either, but there's plenty of it on your menu. Almost all hydrogenated fats contain plenty of the metal, since it is used in the manufacturing process for these substances. You'll find a slug of nickel in margarine, most candies, peanut butter, and solidified cooking fats, among other foods. Too much nickel causes recurrent respiratory infections.

Potassium is an essential metal but it is found in so many foods that it's not really a problem unless you're taking some kind of powerful drug, like a diuretic, that wastes the potassium from your body. In that case you'd be smarter to either cut down on the drug—with your doctor's approval, of course—or increase your intake of foods containing potassium. There are plenty of foods like that, including such ordinary things as bananas and oranges. You can buy potassium pills—they will run about one cent for 40 milligrams of potassium or $120 a pound. You can also eat one little dried apricot, which contains 200 times more potassium than one of those little pills—and as we always say, tastes better.

Are there any more important minerals?

The list of minerals is really a long one but that's just about all the important examples—with one exception: the glamour girl of minerals, the "answer to all your problems," the one and only, last but not least: ZINC!

Zinc? For years zinc was the stuff they put on galvanized iron to keep it from rusting. Now zinc is galvanizing sales of little pink pills. Zinc used to be the stuff we used on the baby's bottom—in the form of zinc oxide —to clear up the diaper rash. Suddenly zinc is very very big in the vitamin-mineral line. Listen to what the ads say:

"Can a deficiency of this mineral vitally affect your health? Research positively says 'yes'! Soil deficient in zinc is found to seriously affect the quality of all the food you eat. Studies reveal the vital role of zinc in protecting important body functions. . . ." And on and on.

Of course, it's stupidity. Every essential vitamin and mineral is, by definition, "essential" to your body. You need them all, and if you had to get them separately in little pills, you would take over 400 pills a day, which wouldn't leave you enough free time to earn the $500 they would cost.

The only ad for zinc pills that's worse than the one quoted is the one that starts "ZINC, the hard-to-get mineral that everybody wants! . . ."

In 1974, the United States alone produced 12 billion pounds of zinc. If old gray zinc is "hard-to-get," we had better find out who's gobbling 12 billion pounds a year. In spite of zinc's "scarcity," that same company will sell you as much as you want for the usual penny-a-pill. They give you 10 tiny milligrams for that amount; they are socking you $480 a pound. With one phone call you can buy up to a million pounds of zinc at 37 *cents* a pound. Or you can save the price of the phone call and just eat protein foods, whole grain cereals, bran, and pumpkin seeds.

Zinc does play an important role in enzyme functions of the body—like almost everything else you eat. There are about two grams of zinc stored in your body—and in the strangest places. You'll find it in your eyes, toenails,

86

pancreas, white blood cells—and in the case of gentlemen, in the prostate gland.

That's the story of minerals. You need them and you'll get them—if you just eat fresh, wholesome, unprocessed food. It's that simple.

CHAPTER VI
Fat—Part One

Is it true that the American diet contains too much fat?

That depends on what you mean by "too much." The diet of the average American *contains more fat than anything else.* As of now, we consume over 40 percent of our calories each day in plain and fancy fat. Other nations are happier and healthier on much lower fat consumption. Japanese, for example, get only about 10 percent of their daily calories from grease and oil. (Not by coincidence the rate of heart attacks in Japan is also one tenth the U.S. rate.) The typical American sloshes about 100 pounds of fat into his digestive system each year.*

But how can anyone eat that much fat?

It's easy if you don't think about it. Fat is part of the American culture. Flip through the average ladies' magazines or the food section of your newspaper; most of the ads and the recipes are for foods that are basically fat. These are the high-prestige, high-status foods of our society. Every festive occasion in American life floats on fat. Hard to believe? Well, let's look at a sample menu.

How about a nice dinner for the boss or some important

* *Dietary Levels of Households in the U.S.* Washington, D.C., USDA Report #8, 1955.

business contacts? Here we go (the numbers in parentheses indicate the percentage of calories contributed by fat in each item):

Cocktails with cream cheese dip (91% fat) and potato chips (63% fat)
Appetizer: Avocado (90% fat) with mayonnaise (100% fat)
Main course: Porterhouse steak (82% fat) with butter (100% fat)
Vegetables: French-fried potatoes (44% fat)
Salad: Lettuce (0% fat) with "Italian dressing" (97% fat)
Dessert: Old-fashioned pound cake (56% fat) with ice cream (65% fat)

That average "company dinner" runs an average of 79 percent fat (not including the lettuce) and clobbers each diner with *over 5000 calories.* (Remember that every ounce of fat contains 250 percent more calories than an ounce of protein or carbohydrate.)

But that's a special company dinner—how about a more routine meal?

Like breakfast, for instance? Fine. Here goes:

Bacon (77% fat) and fried eggs (72% fat)
Pancakes (41% fat) with butter (100% fat)
Coffee (0% fat) with cream (78% fat)

That adds up to an average of 73 percent fat (not including the coffee, of course) and a calorie load of *over 2000 calories.* And remember we've left out the sweet rolls and a lot of the other high-fat possibilities.

But isn't fat essential in the human diet?

Technically, fat *is* essential, but even the National Research Council only recommends a mere 1 percent of your calories in the form of fat. That adds up to no more than about 30 calories a day—about the amount in *a half teaspoonful* or less of any kind of fat. Some nutrition books make a big point about "essential fatty acids," even going so far as to christen them "vitamin F"—presumably "F for fat." But there's nothing so exotic about a fatty acid, as we will see.

What is a fatty acid?

A fat—any fat—is made up of two substances: *glycerin,* as in cough drops, face cream, and suppositories, and *fatty acids.* There are about two dozen fatty acids, and the number and kinds of fatty acids that are combined with glycerin determine what kind of fat it is that you eat. Research costing millions of dollars has proved that there are three essential fatty acids—fatty acids that your body doesn't make and you can't get along without. During his days in medical school (first-year biochemistry, remember, old buddy?) every doctor learned that the essential fatty acids are *linoleic, linolenic,* and *arachidonic.* There's only one little problem: what they taught us in medical school —and are still teaching as you read these words—is *wrong.* It turns out that your body *does* make arachidonic acid from linoleic. It also turns out that you probably don't need linolenic acid very much. But that's really beside the point: if you consume your half teaspoon a day of soybean oil, corn oil, sunflower oil, cottonseed oil, peanut oil, or almost any of the cheap (*before* they get on the supermarket shelf) vegetable oils, you'll get plenty of the so-called essential fatty acids. But you'll also get them if you just switch to real whole wheat bread instead of the imitation white stuff—these fatty acids are abundant in wheat germ. And you can get them from *any kind of fat:*

butter, lard, bacon grease, chocolate, camel's milk and buffalo fat all supply more than you need.

But what if you don't get enough of these essential fatty acids?

Then brace yourself. You *might*—nobody can predict with certainty—be in for a bad siege of dandruff! You even get clobbered with an attack of brittle hair complicated by split ends! The whole business is a joke—albeit a high-priced joke for the consumer. No one has ever been known to have a deficiency of the three (or is it two?) essential fatty acids unless they had a serious disease that interfered with the fat metabolism of their entire body. Then they could drink a bathtub full of fat and it wouldn't do them one bit of good. When it comes to fat there's only one piece of advice that makes medical and scientific sense: *eat less of it.* The more fat you eliminate from your diet, the healthier you will be, the more attractive you will be (fat isn't sexy), and the longer you are likely to live. You'll also have a lot more money to live on, because fat is the most expensive component of your diet.

How come fat is so expensive?

Because most everyone in our society is standing in line for his daily fat transfusion. Porterhouse steak will cost you about $2.00 a pound—for the whole package: meat, bone, and *fat.* You're paying $2.00 a pound for the 82 percent (calorie basis) fat—the same fat your friendly butcher would probably give you for nothing if you asked nicely. Have you noticed that as the price goes up, more and more of the fat stays on the steak when it goes on the scale? Fat is the great equalizer—for the seller. Sausage-makers dump over 80 percent fat into hot dogs (and other sausages) because they know you'll buy them anyway if the kids cry loud enough. Some inspired hot dog stands even sell the "imitation hot dog"—a concoction that contains nearly 100 percent fat and no meat! It's oodles of fat, a little cornmeal (to keep the grease from running out the ends)—and "artificial meat flavoring." Wow!

Fat has another quality. It adds what food engineers (that's true, they really call themselves "food *engineers*" now) refer to as "richness" and "body." Take commercial white imitation bread, for example. Since it is made with starchy ultrarefined white flour, it has an awful pasty consistency. But if you add cheap coconut oil to the dough, suddenly the bread comes through as "rich" and "moist." It's the same with supermarket bakery products, boxed cake mixes, and even that favorite of the astronauts, powdered imitation orange juice. Without added fat, it would taste like moon gravel mixed with rocket fuel. Even chewing gum gets a shot of grease to give it—get ready!—better "Mouth Feel." What a nifty vocabulary those "food engineers" have.

There's also the prestige angle of fat. Most meat sold in the United States is graded, presumably according to quality but actually according to fat content. There are three grades of beef that consumers generally see: Prime, Choice, and Good. (Actually Prime grade rarely gets into the supermarkets anymore, so let's just make the comparison between Choice and Good.) The number one difference between a *Choice-graded* carcass and a *Good-graded* carcass is the *fat*. The Choice carcass has over *60 percent* more fat than the Good carcass. Choice beef has so much fat that about a fifth of it has to be trimmed off—even the boldest butcher doesn't dare stick you with a steak that has a four-inch frame of fat around it. That fat adds up to about 3 billion pounds every year—which according to the U.S. Department of Agriculture means about $3 billion wasted in putting the fat on the cows, shipping it around, removing it, and disposing of it. But who wants something that's just "Good" when for a few more dimes (not pennies anymore) they can get something that's "Choice"?

It almost seems as if we aren't happy unless we are gobbling something greasy with the fat dripping down from both sides of our mouths. Take the cheeseburger—a fast-food favorite. The "burger" part is about 85 percent fat, the "cheese" part is 73 percent fat, the "sauce" is about 90 percent fat (cheap salad dressing), and even the

93

awful cottony bun has its individual fat content. The french-fried potatoes add their share, shrimp-in-a-basket might as well be shrimp-in-an-oil-drum, fried chicken has more fat than chicken (51 percent fat), and we already know about those greeeaaat hot dogs. Let's check the kid's lunchbox: a simple sandwich with sandwich spread—a mere 86 percent fat. What is delicately termed "luncheon meat" weighs in at 84 percent fat; the butter or mayonnaise that makes it barely palatable is, of course, 100 percent grease.

How about that old favorite—peanut butter, say, one of the "nationally advertised brands"? That contains peanuts, salt, cheap vegetable oil, and refined sugar. It checks out at over 77 percent fat. (For a better diet that will increase the chances of your kids living long enough to grow up, see Chapter XI.)

But aren't some kinds of fats better for you than other kinds?

I was hoping you would ask. We are now about to enter the hall-of-mirrors-now-you-see-it-now-you-don't land of saturates, polyunsaturates, cholesterol, and saturation ratios. It's going to be an interesting trip, and by the time you finish you'll be mad, sad, glad, and ready to punch your friendly food processor right in one of his beady little eyes. You won't be too happy with your local medical society, your federal government, and your American Heart Association. You'll even be a little mad at yourself for being so dumb. But don't get mad at me—I'm just going to tell you what every doctor knows—it's all right there in the medical journals and the textbooks for all of us to read.

Now to business. We've already seen that fats are really composed of two substances: glycerin and fatty acids. The glycerin remains constant, but the kind and proportion of fatty acids are different in each fat. For example, beef fat has a different fatty acid "profile" than olive oil. Butter has a different collection of fatty acids than goose grease.

In every society people have always tended to use the

fat that was cheapest and most abundant. In the United States the grease of choice has traditionally been pork fat, otherwise known as lard. We kill a lot of pigs, pigs are fat, and we've made good use of that valuable food product. Three generations of Americans have fried their food in lard, baked their pies and cakes with lard, and even spread lard on their morning toast.

Spread lard on their morning toast?

Sure—and millions of Americans still do. Check the label on that bargain margarine you find on sale at the supermarket. Odds are that it's mostly lard—but, as we'll see in a couple of more pages, it isn't any worse for you than the unsaturated margarine they hawk on those $100,000-a-minute TV commercials.

But let's get back to fatty acids. There are three key words in understanding what fats are all about: *saturated, unsaturated,* and *polyunsaturated.* You've seen and heard them many times in advertising pitches: "Lower in saturated fats than any other brand tested!" "Supplies the vital polyunsaturates needed to protect your health!" And all the rest. *Polyunsaturated* has gradually become a virtue and *saturated* has become a curse. But it isn't that way at all.

Fatty acids consist basically of carbon atoms, oxygen atoms, and hydrogen atoms. The physical structure of these chemicals is in the form of a cross with the carbon atom at the center and, say, four hydrogen atoms around it, one at each point of the compass. It can look something like this:

$$
\begin{array}{c}
\text{H} \\
| \\
\text{H---C---H} \\
| \\
\text{H}
\end{array}
$$
(In chemist's shorthand, C stands for "carbon"

and H stands for "hydrogen.")

When a carbon atom is hooked to all the hydrogens it can take (four), it is considered *saturated* with hydrogen atoms, as a sponge that can't absorb any more water is considered *saturated* with water. If the carbon atoms of a particular fatty acid can take up a few more hydrogen atoms, it is called *polyunsaturated*. That's it—simple, dull, and very insignificant.

Then why do you see so much advertising about how much better it is to use polyunsaturated fats and oils than the "regular" kind?

The complete answer can be found in one little word: MONEY. You see, you really can't make big money selling fats like lard and butter. Both of those foods are by-products and you can't control the supply. If a lot of pigs are slaughtered and a lot of cows are milked, you end up with a lot of lard and a lot of butter to sell. Government price supports help—that means the government buys butter from the farmers at high prices (paid for by your taxes), then stores it in caves to make butter scarce and keep the price up. After a while the butter gets rancid, so your government usually gives it away to countries like India. (Indians don't use much butter, but they convert it to a clarified butter oil called *ghee*.) It's a good program since it means more money for the companies in the dairy business and also keeps the cost of food low for India. That helps India work on more exciting projects like making nuclear bombs. But what the fat processors really needed was some way to sell cheap everyday chemicals for a premium price—like vitamins. They needed to make the greasy liquids they sell take on a special charisma—like maybe some kind of lifesaving medicine. And strangely enough they opened up a whole new dimension of profit by popping the cork on the greatest swindle in the history of nutrition: CHOLESTEROL!

What is cholesterol?

That's a very interesting question. Everybody who reads the papers or watches television knows the following details about cholesterol:

1. Cholesterol is some kind of fat.
2. You get all your cholesterol from the food you eat.
3. Cholesterol causes heart attacks.
4. A really healthy diet has no cholesterol.

There's only one little problem: *all four statements are sheer nonsense.* Here's the truth:

1. Cholesterol is *not* a fat. It is an *alcohol* in solid form very similar to plain old glycerin.
2. You manufacture within your body, every day, *three times as much* cholesterol as you can possibly consume in your diet.
3. About 80 percent of patients with heart attacks have normal blood cholesterol levels.
4. Cholesterol is an essential part of human metabolism. If you don't know enough to include it in your diet, your body is compelled to manufacture it for you.

The chemical formula for cholesterol is $C_{27}H_{45}OH$, and if you were able in some magical way to get rid of all your cholesterol, as the margarine ads suggest you should, you'd be a goner. Cholesterol is absolutely essential for survival. It must be present in *all* body tissues, and it is especially vital in the brain, spinal cord, nerves, liver, and blood. It is a basic part of bile, vitamin D, cortisone—and *sex hormones*. No cholesterol, no sex! If the weird hate-cholesterol campaign were not so profitable, the fat producers surely would have gone the other way. The National Dairy Council would be running full-page ads shrieking: "Safflower is for wallflowers! Fry everything in butter today and swing tonight!" The health-food magazines would be full of ads like this:

"Beware of cholesterol deficiency! Science has proved that this organic sterol is essential for a normal sex life! *Our* cholesterol is 100 percent natural, extracted from the belly fat of choicest Georgia swine. Each glistening lard capsule is guaranteed to contain twice the minimum daily requirement as established by the National Research Council!"

That's not as strange as it might seem. Up until 1962

the average daily dose of cholesterol was established at 200 to 300 milligrams by medical authorities.*

Should you *really* eat cholesterol?

If you don't want to get sick, *you better eat cholesterol.* Consider the undisputed scientific facts:

The average American eats about 600 milligrams of cholesterol daily. About 300 mg of that is absorbed, and the body manufactures, on its own, another 1000 mg of the solid alcohol. That cholesterol is made in the liver, skin, adrenal glands, intestines, aorta, and testicles. Cholesterol is so vital to your survival that if you don't consume any cholesterol in your diet your dozen little cholesterol factories cook it up out of fat, protein, or carbohydrate. So reducing your cholesterol level is a hopeless struggle.

Why is it hopeless?

For several reasons. First, there is a "cholesterol thermostat" in your body. The chemical is so essential that the less you eat, the more you manufacture, keeping the body supply adequate. The more you eat, the less you produce inside, since you have enough for your daily needs.

Second, the amount of cholesterol you eat doesn't have anything to do with heart attacks. Even the U.S. government insists on that. The Federal Trade Commission forbids anyone to claim that their low-cholesterol, polyunsaturated, gimmicked-up food will prevent a heart attack. (We'll see later on how the oil merchants get around that neatly.)

The whole cholesterol phobia—and that's what it is, a collective obsession with an imaginary danger—got its start in 1911. And the Russians were to blame!

---

* *Taber's Cyclopedic Medical Dictionary.* Philadelphia, F. A. Davis Co., 1962, p. C–51.

The Russians?

Yes, but it was the capitalistic Russians. Dr. Nikolai Anitschkov did a lot of examinations of the arteries of people who had died of heart attacks, and guess what he found? *Cholesterol deposits in the blood vessels.* In those early days of modern medicine, Dr. Anitschkov leaped to the conclusion that the cholesterol you ate all ran into your arteries, clogged them up like sewer pipes, and made your heart stop beating. But the good doctor (and many doctors after him) also found protein, calcium, and vitamin A in the arteries of heart attack victims. Why not start a campaign to eliminate those from your diet? Well, there are a lot of reasons but only one really good one.

What's that good one?

Money, *again.* Selling protein—in the form of meat and chicken—is a multibillion-dollar business in the United States. Peddling calcium (for "strong bones") is a foundation of the very profitable multibillion-dollar milk business. Vitamin A is a nice profitable vitamin. *But nobody makes a penny selling cholesterol.*

The next step took place about 1924 when other myopic scientists started feeding pure cholesterol in the form of crystals to caged rabbits in a laboratory. Can you guess what happened? The poor bunnies developed massive deposits of cholesterol in their little bunny arteries and died. Then the rabbit experts concluded: "If you feed a rabbit a lot of cholesterol, it will get clogged arteries and die." They were 100 percent right, since they were only describing what they had observed. Then they closed their eyes, took a deep breath, and made the big leap: "If people eat cholesterol, they will get clogged arteries and die." They only overlooked one little detail.

What was that?

People aren't bunnies. That's the logical defect in their reasoning—and the reasoning of many scientists today is based on this error. People who die from heart attacks have cholesterol (and other things) in their arteries. Feeding rabbits cholesterol gives them cholesterol in their arteries. But that doesn't mean that feeding people cholesterol gives them heart attacks.

There are plenty of good reasons for that. First, rabbits and humans have completely different digestive systems. Rabbits are vegetarians—a starving cottontail wouldn't even nibble at a sizzling steak. *Rabbits lack any digestive mechanism whatsoever for dealing with cholesterol.* Actually you could live better on rabbit feed than a bunny could survive on your fatty carnivorous diet. They are the worst animals of all to use as a comparison with human beings and were chosen for cholesterol experiments only because they are cheap and have big blood vessels which make them easy to examine after they are killed.

One example of how different rabbits are physically from man is the way they deal with vitamin A. Every morning about 2 A.M., rabbits get up and eat their feces from the day before to absorb the vitamin A they cannot manufacture. (Then they blissfully go back to sleep.) When you start doing that, you can worry about the amount of cholesterol you are eating.

The other defect in the "cholesterol experiments" is that the rabbits are fed pure crystalline cholesterol—the kind available only in a chemical lab at exorbitant cost. Every cholesterol-containing food found in nature also contains a substance known as *lecithin.* And that makes all the difference in the world.

Why is lecithin so important?

Because lecithin is an emulsifier. Cholesterol will not dissolve easily in water, so pure cholesterol does not stay dissolved in a watery solution like human blood. But lecithin
100

has the ability to make cholesterol very easy to dissolve in blood, so it doesn't drop out of solution and build up in the blood vessels of the body. (You can illustrate the principle in your kitchen, if you want to. Put some cold water in a jar—representing blood. Add some cooking oil—representing cholesterol. Notice that they form two separate layers: oil and water don't mix. Cholesterol and blood don't mix. Add a little laundry detergent—an excellent emulsifier. Cover the jar and shake well. The two, oil and water—cholesterol and blood—should mix nicely because the emulsifier brings them together and keeps them there.) So, in The Great Scheme of Things you have been amply protected from the "hazards" of cholesterol by the fact that all natural cholesterol-containing foods (but not all processed foods) have plenty of lecithin to keep the cholesterol from making trouble. To put it in other terms, lecithin keeps cholesterol honest.

Then shouldn't we take extra lecithin?

You can if you want to. A 260-milligram lecithin capsule will run you about one cent—that adds up to about $20 a pound. Considering that lecithin is a waste product of soybean processing and can be bought wholesale for about 20 cents a pound, you might as well buy caviar—which incidentally tastes much better than lecithin and attracts a better class of dinner partner. You will find plenty of lecithin in your diet—enough to emulsify more cholesterol than you could possibly eat. It is also added as a preservative to most cooking oils, and you'll find it in chocolate, mayonnaise, margarine, and ice cream. (Incidentally its presence in chocolate works against you.)

Anyway, the cholesterol phobia soon began to ring bells at the cash register.

How come?

Well, two things happened. The American Medical Association, the American Heart Association, and a lot of other official-sounding groups that should know better began to spread the word that you shouldn't eat "cholesterol." That got into the ladies' magazines, the newspapers, and television. Then someone came up with the exciting discovery that you could "lower your blood cholesterol level" by changing the kind of fat you ate in your diet! Wow!

Let's stop a moment and check the figures. There are 220 million Americans, each consuming an average of 100 pounds of fat a year. That's 21.5 billion pounds of fat yearly. If you sell them pig fat at 5 cents a pound profit, that's a piddling $1 billion profit. But sell them expensive "unsaturated" fats at, say, 25 cents a pound profit, that's over *$5 billion profit*. Begin to get the idea? (Incidentally the fat processors will insist that they don't make anything like *that* kind of profit. I can hear it now: "Our adjusted net profits are only 1.3 percent of average annual gross sales, adjusted." Do the calculation yourself. Check your newspaper for the wholesale price of corn oil per pound. Then check the price per pint at your supermarket. Two cups of oil weigh about one pound. See what I mean?)

The so-called low-cholesterol diet that is pounded into your head twenty-four hours a day is a ticket to the poorhouse, a chance to make yourself sick, and the perfect way to look like a dummy—and a prune-faced dummy at that, as we'll see in the next chapter.

Why is the low-cholesterol diet so dumb?

Let's see what it consists of. According to the cholesterol "theory," you are supposed to eat *in limited quantities*, if at all, the following nourishing foods: (1) eggs, (2) meat, (3) whole milk, (4) cheese, (5) butter, (6) shrimp, (7) lobster, (8) olive oil and peanut oil.

You are supposed to substitute low-fat milk for whole milk, corn oil margarine for butter, some yucky imitation egg product for nice fresh eggs, and even imitation powdered "coffee whitener" for a little shot of milk in your coffee. That advice is reinforced by the threat of an imminent heart attack if you dare to put a little bit of butter

.on your pancakes. Even your family doctor is likely to tell you—sincerely—"It's better if you don't have more than one egg a week." Of course, he means well but he really doesn't know why he's saying it. Eggs are supposed to be bad, and he doesn't want you to eat anything bad.

Well, aren't eggs bad for you?

No, eggs are good for you. For some reason everyone is on a "hate-eggs" kick. Even federal judges are hating eggs.

In the August 9, 1976, *Wall Street Journal* there is a hair-raising story of how "a federal court in Chicago" ordered a group called "The National Commission on Egg Nutrition" (obviously an egg-sellers association) to stop saying that eating eggs doesn't increase the risk of heart attacks. The judges pointed out: "Numerous medical investigators have linked high cholesterol intake in food to high cholesterol levels in the blood." Yippee! The next move should be to declare all the hens in the country in contempt of court and make the possession, use, or sale of eggs a felony.

You mean the judges were wrong?

The current informed medical consensus can be summarized as follows:

"The level of cholesterol in the blood is not significantly influenced by the amount present in foods. By omitting protective foods such as eggs, milk, and organ meats from the diet, one may be denying the body needed protein, minerals and vitamins."

Back in 1968, a leading medical journal called *Metabolism* published the results of a fascinating little project done with two groups of people. Half the subjects were confined to bed because they were sick, and the other half were normal people like the rest of us. All the participants were given the equivalent of nine eggs a day—more than the average person eats, to be sure. At the end of the study period only two of the sick people showed any elevation in cholesterol—and they'd had trouble in that area before. After eating their nine eggs every day, the healthy people had lower cholesterol than when they started. Judge for yourself!*

In addition, eggs have plenty of lecithin to emulsify the cholesterol that you so desperately need. Now before we go on to show how the "low-cholesterol" diet can give you heart attacks, cancer, and make pretty girls look old and ugly, let's review the gospel of saturated-unsaturated fats once again quickly.

According to the questionable theory, if you increase the amount of polyunsaturated fat in your diet, and decrease the amount of saturated fat, you will lower your blood cholesterol level. That, in turn, will decrease the amount of cholesterol deposited in your arteries, which will reduce your chances of getting a heart attack—or so the story goes. In all fairness, it's a very attractive tale—it makes the incredibly complex metabolism of the human body simple and understandable and reduces the whole problem of heart attacks to grease clogging your sink. Shoot in some Drano in the form of unsaturated fats, and you're out of danger.

But unfortunately the whole folklore of saturated-unsaturated fats just doesn't hold together. Look at the facts and make up your own mind.

What are the facts?

For an answer to that question, just turn the page and plunge into the next chapter.

---

* Incidentally about one out of every thousand Americans has a condition called *Type IV lipidemia*, which is a hereditary inability to metabolize cholesterol. They *do* have elevated cholesterol levels if they consume a reasonable amount of cholesterol. But we all don't have to change our diet just because of the misfortune of one tenth of one percent of the population. *Or do we?*

CHAPTER VII
Fat—Part Two

What are the facts about *unsaturated* and *saturated* fats?

The facts are these: fats with a high degree of *unsaturated fats* include corn oil, safflower oil, soybean oil, cottonseed oil and some other seed oils. Butter has a relatively low concentration of *unsaturated fat*. Therefore your doctor—and television and magazine ads—tell you to substitute corn oil margarine for butter to lower your cholesterol and avoid heart attacks.

Remember exactly what those ads say? One of my favorites is the following:

The picture is a big bowl of peas with a big greasy chunk of margarine on top. But wait—the margarine is in the form of "Rx." Get it? This fatty, artificially colored, artificially flavored yellow stuff is really medicine—and it's worth the big price tag. The headline says: "X is the margarine most recommended by doctors! . . . Twice as many doctors recommended and personally used X margarine as any other brand." What does this mean to you?

Not much. A margarine company can send out 300,000 free coupons to doctors to make sure they can say that the MDs use their brand. Wouldn't you use a food product if it came to you free? But let's go on. Watch how the truth slips in from time to time:

"No margarine alone can reduce serum cholesterol. Any doctor will tell you that. But used in a total dietary program . . . along with lean meats, fewer eggs [there's the hate-egg campaign again], and skim milk, X margarine can help reduce serum cholesterol. Up to 17 percent in clinical tests."

Let's translate that into English. They are saying that margarine won't lower your cholesterol, but if you change your diet, in spite of eating their imitation butter your blood cholesterol will go down a whole 17 percent. I will now make a better claim. Eat whatever you want—including hyena fat if you like it—but every night at bedtime, put your hand on this book and say: "Good-bye, cholesterol." Take a cholesterol test every week for four weeks, and you will find that at some point your cholesterol will go down at least 10 percent and maybe even more.

You're kidding! It can't work that way, can it?

It sure can. The cholesterol-exploiters know a few medical facts that they aren't telling you—and they use that partial knowledge to scare you into buying their overpriced inferior products. That's right—inferior. Just read the label on that expensive margarine carefully:

"Partly hydrogenated soybean oil and coconut oil, water, salt, vegetable mono and diglycerides, lecithin, benzoate of soda, artificially flavored and artificially colored, vit. A (palmitate), vit. D. calciferol."

That's a combination straight out of Junior's chemistry set—and it's made by the tank-carload in big factories. Butter, for better or worse, is a natural food product made by a cow. People have been eating butter for 50,000 years —long before anyone had the first recognized heart attack in about 1910. People have been eating imitation butter called "margarine" less than 75 years—as the incidence of heart attack soars.

Anyhow this is the way the cholesterol-margarine swindle works. No medical lab in the world will get exactly the same value for blood cholesterol in the same person on two different days—or even at different hours on the same day. There are two reasons for this. First, the test itself is not that accurate—there can be a 10 percent variation in the results simply because of the way the test chemicals react. Second—and they never tell you this in the ads—your blood cholesterol level (and that includes other related measurements like total lipids, triglycerides, etc.) is not anchored at a fixed point. During the day it can vary as much as 20 percent up or down. Take a cholesterol test after a big fatty meal and it's up. Jog a mile before breakfast in the morning and your cholesterol level can be 20 percent *lower.* The margarine peddlers know that—but they don't think that *you* do. Besides, they hedge their bet by saying, "Lowers cholesterol *up to* 17 percent." Obviously that doesn't mean "lowers cholesterol 17 percent." So take 1000 people, feed them X brand of imitation butter. Even if the cholesterol in 999 of them goes up on that greasy kid stuff, as long as *one* cholesterol test in *one* person is lower by 17 percent, you can run the ad, make the claim, and sell a million dollars' worth of overpriced chemistry-set imitation butter.

If that's true, why don't people know about it?

It is true—and at least *you* know about it now. But there is no money to be made by telling the whole story. They tell you enough to scare you down to the supermarket.

There are four other aspects of the "cholesterol controversy" that you should know about as well. The enemies of cholesterol constantly remind us—in their ads and in the medical "research" they finance—that we must consume *unsaturated* fats to lower our blood cholesterol. All their advertising for margarine hits one point over and over again: their product contains *polyunsaturated oils.* One margarine factory goes so far as to insist that their imitation butter contains "pure liquid polyunsaturated oil." Good luck.

Good luck to whom?

To the poor folks who think they are getting polyunsaturated oils in their artificially colored, artificially flavored little bars of shortening. There's one key question that has to be answered—how did all that wonderful "pure *liquid* polyunsaturated oil" turn into a *solid* bar of margarine? It happens like this:

In the presence of metallic nickel, hydrogen gas is bubbled through a tank of "pure liquid polyunsaturated oil." The hydrogen causes the liquid fat to solidify, so that it can be formed into bars of margarine. (It also deposits a certain amount of nickel in the finished product, which is not necessarily beneficial to your health.)

That process is called, understandably, *hydrogenation.* Besides hardening cheap vegetable fats, hydrogenation does two other things. First, it converts *polyunsaturated* fats into *saturated* fats. What that means is you are paying big money for *polyunsaturated* margarine but what you are getting is a product that offers just the opposite. Let's check the textbooks:

"The common sources of *saturated* fats are *hydrogenated shortenings,* butter, lard, coconut oil, and animal fat."*

Understand that clearly. In the process of making liquid corn oil, safflower oil, and all the other "polyunsaturated" oils into margarine, they are transformed into plain ordinary "saturated" oils. That has to be one of the greatest unexposed scandals in history. By hardening the vegetable oils, the margarine sellers are offering you the very *saturated* fats they claim to be helping you avoid. That's not too exciting, is it? It means, of course, that you are paying for polyunsaturates and getting all the advantages of lard —except for the lower price.

And there's a second little fact that they keep out of the $100,000-a-minute TV commercials.

---

* Krause, Marie, *Food, Nutrition, and Diet Therapy.* Philadelphia, W. B. Saunders, 1969, and McOsker, D. E., et al., The influence of partially hydrogenated dietary fats on serum cholesterol levels. *J.A.M.A.,* 180:380, 1962.

What's that?

Simply this. The same polyunsaturated fat can actually exist in two forms according to the way its molecules are arranged. Chemists call these two forms *cis* and *trans*. In nature, most polyunsaturated fats occur in the *cis* form. However, the *trans* form of polyunsaturated fats is found in beef fat (as well as in the fat of some other animals). As any dedicated reader of the anticholesterol pamphlets knows, beef fat is a no-no: "Carefully trim the fat from your steak before eating it to lower your cholesterol intake."

But if you hydrogenate polyunsaturated oils to make them into margarine, you change the *cis* form into the *trans* form—and you might as well cut the fat off your steak and spread it on your toast in the morning.*

The margarines that claim to contain liquid polyunsaturated oil may have, technically, contained liquid oil at one time—but when you peel back that fancy foil wrapping you will observe that all the liquid has been solidified in the process of changing unsaturated into saturated.

Then what's the conclusion?

The conclusion is this: If you still believe that eating polyunsaturated fats will help you avoid a heart attack, one of the worst and most expensive sources of those fats, according to responsible medical researchers, is margarine.

There's another fascinating little myth in the folklore of cholesterol. That's the one that says unsaturated fats have a "protective effect" against the cholesterol-raising influence of saturated fats. For example, you're supposed to be able to keep a big steak from elevating your blood cholesterol level if you eat some of that unsaturated margarine along with it. Sounds great—eat all that "bad stuff" and then wash away the effects with "good stuff." Let's look at the calculations:

---

* Berk, Z., *Introduction to the Biochemistry of Food*. Amsterdam, Oxford, New York, Elsevier Publishing Co., 1976, p. 172.

According to the cholesterol-counters, if you eat an 8-ounce steak, you can undo the "bad" effects by smothering it in 12 ounces of unsaturated margarine. Great for margarine sales, but look what it does to you. The steak plus the margarine comes out to 3250 calories. That means the entire meal can add up to 5000 big calories to your diet. Try three "protective" meals like that and you'll be gobbling 15,000 calories a day as you float away in grease. Your blood will be replaced by margarine, your weight will level off at 500 pounds, and you will sit at the table in your reinforced dining chair fighting back nausea as you soak your steaks in big bowls of congealed fat.

As a practical matter, if Americans began to consume 150 percent of their meat intake in fat, margarine would have to be delivered to their homes by tanker truck.

But hasn't anybody tested this cholesterol theory to see if it really works?

Sure, you've tested it on yourself and your family. About 200 million Americans have been involuntary guinea pigs as the kind and amount of fat in the American diet have been radically altered in the past thirty years. The final result is absolutely undeniable. Here it is, once and for all: *Changing the fat content of your diet will not decrease the risk of heart attack.*

But what about all the medical research that alleges just the opposite?

That medical research simply doesn't square with the facts. Here they are:

1. Since 1909, Americans have shifted the ratio of unsaturated to saturated fats a gigantic 37 percent—precisely the shift that is supposed to lower the incidence of heart attacks. But since 1909, the incidence of heart attacks among Americans has zoomed into outer space. The death rate from heart disease in 1909 was 153 per 100,000. In 1973 it was 360 per 100,000. If the ratio of unsaturated

to saturated fats in the diet had anything to do with anything, the rate should have gone down.*

2. Just looking at the period from 1949 to 1973, when the sharpest alterations in fat consumption took place, is a shocking experience. Sixty-five percent of all American families stopped using butter, consumption of whole milk and eggs dropped drastically, average fat consumption fell 30 percent, and almost everyone went crazy for so-called "unsaturated fats." If there was ever a golden opportunity to see if changing the amount and kind of fat in the diet would affect death rates from heart attacks, that was it. The death rate from heart attacks certainly did change: *it went up!* In 1949, about 400,000 Americans died of heart attacks. In 1973, about 800,000 perished in the crushing agony of a heart muscle deprived of blood.

Any questions?

But why don't the people who sell the unsaturated oils tell us those things?

Because they are not running a consumer education program—they are dedicated to buying greasy liquids at the lowest possible cost and selling them at the highest possible prices. They tell you the facts that sell you their product—and their motto is what you don't know won't hurt you. But what you don't know just *might* hurt you.

For example, when you fry food in polyunsaturated oils like safflower, corn oil, cottonseed oil, and the rest, strange things happen. At temperatures over 200°F—the temperature in your frying pan is over 400°F—unsaturated oils lose their unsaturation and begin to raise the level of cholesterol in the blood—for whatever that's worth. The big point is that you shouldn't have to pay big money to *raise* your cholesterol. In animal experiments, test animals sicken and die when given food fried in polyunsaturated oils. Those animals given food fried in butter remain nor-

* National Center for Health Statistics, Dept, HEW, U.S. Government, Washington, D.C.

mal and healthy.* Obviously something bad happens to the chemical composition of polyunsaturated oils when they are heated even a little bit. So it's better to fry in butter or olive oil or even pure lard—and if you insist on frying in polyunsaturated oils, be prepared for the unexpected.

You said something about unsaturated oils making people look old and ugly?

Right. A plastic surgeon graded over 1000 women between the ages of 17 and 81 to see whether they looked older than they really were. The results were correlated with the women's diets—and they were amazing! Fully 78 percent of the women who showed signs of premature aging were devotees of the polyunsaturated fat diet. They showed such unexciting signs of early old age as crow's feet, excessive wrinkles, and loss of skin tone.†

There's also another *little* technical detail they don't let you in on. Do you buy safflower oil to get the supposed benefit of "polyunsaturates"? Do you pay a big price for that safflower oil? Are you getting the good safflower oil, or the *other* kind?

You mean there's more than one kind of safflower oil?

Oh, yes. Didn't you know? There is "safflower oil" and "high oleic safflower oil"—and there's a big difference between the two. An interesting way of comparing the amount of unsaturates or polyunsaturates is to measure the amount of linoleic acid in the oil. The more linoleic acid, the greater the degree of polyunsaturation. At the top of that list—most unsaturated—is safflower oil, with a linoleic content of 75 percent. At the bottom of the list are such saturated—and supposedly "bad"—fats as butter with 2 percent linoleic acid.

* Rakel Kurkela et al., *Zusammenfassender Vortrag mit Literaturangaben*, 1968, No. 3, pp. 57–65.
† Pinckney, E. R., *Medical Counterpoint*, Feb. 1973.

So buy safflower oil, even though it's really expensive, and you'll get a high linoleic percentage? No, not exactly, because there's another kind of safflower that looks and smells and tastes exactly the same. It's called "high oleic safflower" and it has barely 10 percent linoleic acid. By that measure it has less polyunsaturated power than plain old pig fat—lard—which checks in at 14 percent linoleic. If it sounds like a consumer gyp, it is. Try asking at the supermarket next time what kind of safflower you're getting for your money. I hope you get an answer.

But that same linoleic acid percentage is also the key to the biggest fat-oil-cholesterol swindle of all time. It's almost exactly equivalent to being sold the Brooklyn Bridge every time you sit down and eat—and occasionally for a between-meal snack.

What's that all about?

This is what it's all about. The very same companies that tell you to avoid even the tiniest drop of saturated fat are slipping you massive amounts of the worst of the saturated fats when they think you aren't looking! It happens like this:

Almost all the major sellers of "polyunsaturated oils"—corn, safflower, soybean, and the rest—have a lot of other products to sell. These include thousands of items ranging from cakes, cookies, and a wide assortment of pastries to coffee "creamers," candy, salad dressings, *margarine,* bread, and many other foods you've already eaten today. Those items contain oil too—plenty of it—and if you want to know what kind it is, just look on the label. It says right there in big letters: "VEGETABLE OIL." Ah yes, but *which* vegetable? The FDA, which is responsible for guarding your health, doesn't *care* if you know; the food processor *doesn't want* you to know. The vegetable from whence that oil comes, my friends, is actually a fruit—none other than the humble *coconut,* swaying in the breeze in exotic tropical climes. Wherever they can get away with it, food processors sock the coconut oil to you for a reason you can guess already: it is cheap, cheap, cheap. It is so cheap that until recently its primary use was . . . well, let the French tell it. This is what *Larousse Gastronomique,* the world's leading reference book on food, says about coconut oil:

"This oil is solid at normal temperatures. It is used in cooking by Africans. In other parts of the world *it is used in the manufacture of soap.*"

It should be added, it is also used in cooking by food manufacturers in the United States, disguised as "vegetable oil." As a matter of fact, not too much soap is made from coconut oil these days because the people who are putting it in your cake mixes, cupcakes, cake frostings and bread have driven the price up. It now sells for an outrageous 32 cents a pound! That's up from about 17 cents a pound only a year ago. You see, the more of those breakfast cakes they turn out, the more "lunch-in-a-can" diet drinks they sell, the more infant formulas they sell, the more the demand for coconut oil increases.

You mean there's coconut oil in baby formulas?

Sure, a company's got to make money. Most of the big-name imitation milks that are given new mothers when they leave the hospital are powdered skim milk and guess what—coconut oil snatched from the clutches of the soap makers. But we'll go into that story in detail later. Back to the coconut oil in your diet. The same company that runs full-page ads like this—"Wishing You a Meal Rich in Everything But Saturated Fat . . ." (Kind of gets you right *here,* doesn't it? Right in your heart?)—is selling you a whole range of other food under different labels chock full of coconut oil which guarantees you thousands of meals abundantly "rich in *saturated* fat."

Is coconut oil really a saturated fat?

Is Kennedy an Irish name? According to its linoleic acid content, coconut oil is the *most saturated of the saturated fats.* It is farther down on the list than even the supposed-

114

ly most diabolical of the demons, *butter* and *lard*. By another scientific yardstick—"relative amount of unsaturated plus polyunsaturated fatty acids"*—good-quality safflower oil has a "number" of 132, indicating a high degree of *unsaturation*. Peanut oil has a number of 98, lard slips to 73, butter is a mere 30, but the coconut oil you've eaten today—or fed your kids or even the new baby in his formula—lies at the bottom at 9.

Is there no justice? The company that begs you to save yourself from a heart attack by eating its greasy "polyunsaturated" imitation butter at a dollar a pound slips you coconut oil in the rest of its product line—which, *according to the identical theory,* will set you up to join the other 2000 Americans who die agonizing deaths every day from heart attacks.

But then what should a person do? What should we eat and feed our families?

All I can tell you is what I do, what I advise my patients, and what I feed my family. The rest is up to you. The human race as we know it has multiplied (when they weren't busy exterminating themselves) for nearly 50,000 years by consuming a natural diet substantially free from chemicals and processing. Moreover, this diet was based on natural taste-choice. Without going into the theory of physiological perception, people selected natural foods which tasted good. Heart attacks—the disease that unsaturated fat is supposed to save you from—only became a significant disease about 70 years ago when people veered away from a natural diet. So the obvious solution is to go back to a free-selection, taste-oriented diet.

* *Food Engineering,* May 1970.

Specifically what kind of diet is that?

Okay, now brace yourself, because it goes against all those phony charts you've seen in the magazine ads and all those deceitful TV commercials:

1. Eat nutritious foods regardless of their fat content but *only in their natural form.*
2. Drink whole milk since it contains only 3.5 percent fat —at the most. The so-called 2 percent skim milk has only 1 percent less fat and is an inferior product.
3. Eat as many eggs as you feel like eating. They contain lecithin to emulsify the cholesterol and can't do you any harm.
4. Use the kind of cooking oil you like the best, but make sure it's free of chemicals and preservatives, which will do you in a lot faster than the theoretical ratio of saturated to unsaturated fats.
5. Remember butter? It's good on toast, great on pancakes, makes super pies and cakes. Start using it if you like the taste. It's been part of the human diet a lot longer than safflower and soybean oil.
6. Don't waste your money on high-priced fats with health claims. Remember that no one takes an ad to tell you how good natural *unprocessed* fats are.
7. Don't buy any product containing hydrogenated oils— you get a less-nutritious food that has been tinkered with unnecessarily.
8. Don't eat any food that has the words "vegetable oil" on the label unless you know *what* vegetable (or fruit) that oil came from. If the company that makes it doesn't tell you what it is, could it be because they don't want you to know?

But don't the most prominent scientists endorse the cholesterol theory of heart attacks?

No one likes to be reminded of this, but it wasn't too many years ago that the most prominent scientists were warning you that night air was poisonous, man would never fly, and the earth was flat. The only difference this time is that some of the richest corporations on earth have found a way to distort the digestive problems of rabbits and use it to scare the daylights out of you. If you want to tune in on the *latest* scientific theory, some researchers now believe that polyunsaturated fats and low-cholesterol diets lower the blood cholesterol level by forcing the cholesterol out of the blood and into the walls of the arteries, where it clogs them up. Think about *that!*

CHAPTER VIII
Carbohydrates

What are carbohydrates?

Try it this way: let's check our knowledge of carbohydrates with the following test. Which of the following statements about carbohydrates are true?

Carbohydrates are:

1. Something bad that will make you fat.
2. An essential part of your diet.
3. Undesirable foods that rot your children's teeth.
4. The fastest route to a heart attack.
5. Good wholesome food.
6. A way to get gypped out of your food dollars.

If you marked *all six correct,* you know a lot more about carbohydrates than the food processors of America think you know. Just as with protein and fat, the gigantic food companies and their play-for-pay experts have done a big number on carbohydrates.

What kind of "number" have they done on carbohydrates?

This one: by means of an intensive advertising campaign they have convinced you that carbohydrates are bad, that they will make you fat, and that you should eliminate them from your diet. Since you have to eat *something,* that means you substitute large amounts of expensive protein and fat for economical and nutritious carbohydrates. That's bad—but even worse is the fact that the same companies that switch you out of good-quality natural carbohydrate switch you into cheap overrefined junk carbohydrate. That's what rots the teeth of your children, makes you fat, pushes you closer and closer to a heart attack, and robs you of the best part of your food dollar.

There are actually three kinds of carbohydrates—two very good kinds and one very bad kind. The good kinds are cheap, tasty and plentiful. The bad kind is expensive to you (cheap to the food companies) and can literally ruin your life. To understand how this all happens, we have to start with a group of chemicals called *monosaccharides.*

What are monosaccharides?

Monosaccharides are the building blocks of carbohydrates. Chemists call them *simple sugars,* but that has nothing to do with their taste, since many of them are not even sweet. Monosaccharides are made up of little particles of carbon, hydrogen, and oxygen, all hooked together—that's why they're called carb-o-hydrates. There are two important types of these simple sugars—*glucose and fructose.*

Glucose occurs naturally in fruits, corn, and honey, and it is also the chemical that your body depends on for mechanical energy. In a sense, it is the gasoline of the human body. When you turn this page, you are using energy derived directly from glucose to do it. Every 100 cc of blood contains about 100 milligrams of glucose. As the glucose is used up, it is instantly replaced from the liver —but more about that in a few pages.

The other monosaccharide, fructose, is found in fruits, vegetables, and honey. (As a matter of fact, it's the fructose that gives honey its characteristic flavor.)

These simple sugars are combined in nature in various forms to make up *disaccharides,* or "double sugars." For example, *glucose* and *fructose* join together to make *sucrose*. *Glucose* and *galactose* mix to form *lactose,* or milk sugar. Sucrose, incidentally, is table sugar, that white stuff you eat by the ton. (The average American will literally eat about 2000 pounds of white sugar over the next 12 years at present consumption rates.) Lactose is the sugar found in human milk—too few Americans ever taste that anymore. (There *are* exceptions, since lactose is also used to adulterate heroin.)

But people can't live on things like white sugar and lactose, can they?

Hardly—although almost the entire population of the United States seems to be trying to survive on that kind of junk. About a third of the current U.S. consumption of carbohydrates is sugar and syrup. That means that the average person, including growing children, has to try to wring a substantial portion of his nutritional needs from worthless refined sugar. If these people would only substitute decent carbohydrates, their lives would be better in every way.

But I always thought that any kind of carbohydrate made you fat? Isn't that true?

That's what they'd like you to believe. The *right kind of carbohydrate* is the single most important element in your diet. It can be the cheapest kind of food you eat, the most nourishing, and the *least* fattening. One of the most obvious tricks played on unsuspecting dieters is the so-called low-carbohydrate diet. The idea is that you can lose weight by eating protein instead of carbohydrate. What the low-carbohydrate hucksters never tell you are the following two scientific facts:

1. *One gram of protein supplies exactly four calories.*
2. *One gram of carbohydrate supplies exactly four calories.*

121

There's no way in the world to get away from those scientific facts.

In practical terms it means that steak and baked potato have exactly the same ability to make you fat. Given the choice between a steak and a baked potato, most experienced dieters would opt for the steak. But let's check the facts: 3½ ounces of porterhouse steak provide 465 calories. Three and a half ounces of baked potato provide 93 calories. That means you can eat *five* average baked potatoes without getting more calories than come pouring out of *one* steak. A standard 12-ounce T-bone steak, even with all the fat trimmed away, socks you with 768 calories. That's the equivalent of almost 2 *pounds* of baked potatoes.

But how come there are so many calories in protein?

Because protein in the form of meat—the way that most Americans eat it—is loaded with fat. And fat makes you fat—fast. If you don't eat plenty of good-quality carbohydrate, you're fooling yourself, driving your food costs through the roof, and hurting your body. There are four very good reasons to eat carbohydrate—and not just a little bit of it:

1. Carbohydrate is absolutely essential to human life. Your blood sugar—or blood glucose—is carbohydrate and directly derived from the carbohydrate that you consume each day. If your blood carbohydrate drops below a minimum level, your brain is starved for carbohydrate and within minutes starts to die.

2. Carbohydrate saves protein. An adequate intake of carbohydrate keeps you healthy on much less protein. That's why the country people of almost every culture in the world instinctively combine carbohydrate with their protein intake in some form or other. In Hawaii it's *poi*, in Mexico *tortillas*, in Europe *bread*, in India *chapati*, and so on. If you eat good-quality unrefined carbohydrate at the same time you consume protein, your body is able to prosper on much less protein.

3. Carbohydrate is essential for the utilization of fats. If

the high fat intake of the American diet doesn't have plenty of carbohydrate to go along with it, dietary fat cannot be burned properly. It's similar to burning wood in a fireplace without enough air; the wood smolders instead of burning and puts out a lot of acrid smoke. Fats that are eaten without enough carbohydrate produce "smoky ashes" called *ketones* that poison the body and produce a potentially fatal condition called *acidosis*.

That incidentally was the basis of an interesting little diet. Every doctor knows that a diet high in fat and low in carbohydrate eventually produces nausea, loss of appetite, and the accumulation of poisonous ketones in the body. In recent years at least two or three doctors have capitalized on this scientific principle by pushing fad diets that were very low in carbohydrate and very high in fat. You've probably seen the ads:

"Lose weight the easy way! All the mayonnaise, fried chicken, ice cream, and french-fried potatoes you can eat! Don't suffer! Get slim while gorging on your favorite rich foods!"

Yes, you can get slim, you can get sick, you can get surgery (especially of the gallbladder), and you might even get dead—on the low-carbohydrate diet.

4. One of the important carbohydrates, lactose, stays in the large intestine a relatively long time and encourages the production there of important substances like vitamin K, niacin, and others.

What's the best way to get carbohydrate in your diet?

By eating foods that are high in good-quality carbohydrate. But that's not as easy as it sounds. Common sources of carbohydrate in the American diet are things like bread, spaghetti, macaroni, rice, potatoes, and fruits and vegetables. Almost without exception they have been systematically stripped of their value as a source of decent nutrition. Two of the primary sources of carbohydrate in the diet of Americans have been reduced to grim jokes. The first joke is called "bread" and the second joke is called "breakfast cereal." Let's take a look at "bread" first.

What's so bad about American bread?

Everything. Once upon a time bread was known as "the staff of life"—a better description of American bread might be "the stuff of lies." Ninety-five percent of the "bread" sold in the United States is a product known as "enriched white bread." It is *not* bread. It is doubtfully *enriched*. It is very definitely *white*.

Let's go back to the origin of the substance known as "bread." Since pre-Biblical times men have been grinding grains of wheat between stones to produce a gritty powder called flour. Those ground-up grains of wheat were mixed with yeast and salt and water to make a dough. The dough was allowed to rise (as a result of the carbon dioxide gas formed by the yeast), and the risen mass was baked in an oven to form bread. That's *bread*. The atrocity that cowers in plastic bags labeled B-R-E-A-D on supermarket shelves *is not bread*.

What do you mean it's not bread? The label says it's bread.

The label is there to make you feel better. This is the way it really is:

A grain of wheat has three components: bran, wheat germ, and endosperm. If you are going to get any real nutritional benefit from bread, you must consume all three components and in the proportion that God put them there. Unfortunately the Divine Plan does not coincide with the greed of flour millers. Insects like to eat bran because their little insect instincts tell them it is good for them. Insects also like to eat wheat germ because it makes them strong and healthy. Flour millers like to store flour for long periods of time so they can buy it cheap and sell it at high prices, and they don't like insects to nibble at their assets. So about eighty years ago they figured out a cheap way to get rid of the bran and the wheat germ in the flour. They simply turn whole wheat flour into white flour. They pass those plump little grains of wheat under high-pressure steel rollers that reduce them to a fine dust.

Then they remove the wheat germ and bran, leaving only the next-to-worthless pale white starchy endosperm. Endosperm keeps almost forever.

Why does the endosperm keep so well?

Because bugs don't eat it. Why don't bugs eat it? Because there isn't enough nutrition in a ton of white flour to keep one teenie-weenie little bug alive. A diet of so-called bread made from white flour—taken right off the supermarket shelves—can't keep laboratory animals alive, and it can't keep your children alive.

There are a couple of other reasons to get rid of the good parts of the wheat grain. The bran makes tiny dark specks in white flour, and it also makes it harder to chew. Americans have been taught to like everything white, and they don't like to chew. Millions of them now have false teeth anyway, having lost their real teeth from a diet of white flour and other nice white overrefined foods.

There's another good reason to make whole wheat flour into white flour—if you're in the milling business. People who raise livestock, especially pigs, know the importance of good nutrition—for their animals, not for themselves. (One of the great tragedies in life is to see a seemingly intelligent farmer order the best possible diet for his pigs, which he raises to die, while he feeds rotten white "bread" to his children, whom he raises, presumably, to live.) So there's a big profitable animal-feed market for bran and the wheat germ which the miller gets free. The best part of the grain of wheat is stolen before it ever gets to you and is poured into animals to make them healthier than American children.

Isn't that an exaggeration?

If you think so, look at the scientific data. When they take the wheat germ and bran out of the flour they sell you —and out of all the products that are made with that flour—the millers are removing the following:

94% of the pyridoxine	27% of the protein	97% of the thiamine
66% of the riboflavin	57% of the pantothenic acid	76% of the iron
74% of the potassium	60% of the calcium	
50% of the linoleic acid	78% of the magnesium	

The millers also rob you of significant amounts of phosphorus, manganese, copper, sulfur, iodine, fluorine, chloride, sodium, silicon, boron, inositol, folic acid, choline, and vitamin E.

There's another interesting point you won't find on the wrapper of your nice white imitation bread. The wheat germ contains a protein that is a complete and excellent-quality protein—as nourishing as a piece of beefsteak. But you'll never see it in your nice cottony slice of white "bread." Even as you sit down to breakfast, the cows and pigs are eating the wheat germ and bran that belong to you. You can, of course, buy them back at up to $1.20 a pound for the bran (in fancy brand-name boxes) and up to $20 a pound for wheat germ capsules. Or you could make your own whole wheat bread. (More about that later.)

But isn't all the white bread that's sold now "enriched"?

Yes, it certainly is. And most of the miserable products made from white flour are also "enriched," like spaghetti, macaroni, cakes, cookies, pies, gravies, waffles, cake mixes, pancake mixes and all the rest of the instant mixes that clog the grocery shelves. But that's not good—that's *BAD*. It's bad because it makes you think white bread and white flour and the junk made from them are decent and wholesome. "Enriched" is a wonderful word designed to instill confidence in a product. After all, whole wheat flour isn't "enriched," is it? It doesn't have to be—it has everything you need already in it.

In the process of milling, over 26 essential elements are totally or partially removed from the flour. The laughable process of "enrichment" puts back about one sixth of a cent worth of cheap synthetic vitamins consisting of thiamine, riboflavin, and niacin. They also dump in a little tiny bit of iron, often in the form of iron filings. If someone pulled 26 of your teeth and gave you four little false teeth in return, would you consider your mouth to have been "enriched"?

But at least "enrichment" shows that the food industry cares about the consumer, doesn't it?

Not if you know the whole story it doesn't. That rotten white bread and white flour wasn't enriched in the United States until 1939 when World War II was about to explode upon us. It was the generals and the admirals who insisted on "enriching" the bread and flour out of fear that their soldiers wouldn't be able to stand up to the whole-grain-eating Germans and Japanese. And the box score for "enriched" flour tells the story:

Whole Wheat Flour		*"Enriched" White Flour*
1.1 mg	Pantothenic acid (a B-complex vitamin)	0.465 mg
0.34 mg	Vitamin B_6	0.06 mg
4.3 mg	Niacin*	3.5 mg
0.12 mg	Riboflavin*	0.26 mg
0.55 mg	Thiamine* (Vitamin B_1)	0.44 mg
113 mg	Magnesium	25 mg
370 mg	Potassium	95 mg
3.3 mg	Iron*	16 mg
41 mg	Calcium*	2.9 mg
2.3 grams	Fiber	0.3 grams
13.3 grams	Protein	10.5 grams

In spite of the highly touted "enrichment," unenriched whole wheat flour contains more of every valuable ingredient with the exception of riboflavin. It is worth noting

* Added to white flour to enrich it. Calcium is only required for self-rising flour and self-rising cornmeal.

that the riboflavin in "enriched" products is synthetic and the riboflavin in whole wheat flour is natural. Which would you rather have, if you had the choice?

But there are also a few other things in your imitation white bread that you won't read on the label.

What are those? And by the way, why do you keep calling it *"imitation white bread"?*

Let's take the last question first. Bread is whole grain flour, water, salt, and yeast. The stuff you're eating and giving to your growing children is a bizarre combination of artificial chemicals that only helps the bread peddlers —and can hurt you. There's a little gimmick that the food companies love, the FDA allows, and you've probably never heard about. It's called a "standard of identity." Once the food manufacturers and the FDA agree on what can go into a food product, the list of items goes into a dusty government file instead of on the label. (If you want to look it up for yourself, check the Code of Federal Regulations, Title 21, parts 10 through 85. That's one book you won't find at your supermarket check-out counter.) So your loaf of imitation white bread, dutifully "enriched," can contain some or all of the following chemicals and exotic substances: monoglycerides and diglycerides, diacetyl tartaric acid, propylene glycol, carrageenin, rice flour, potato starch, ground soybeans, calcium lactate, ammonium phosphate, calcium bromate, azodicarbonamide, sodium stearoyl-2-lactylate, polysorbate 60, and plaster of Paris.

Hold on a minute. Did you say *plaster of Paris?*

Sure. Are you surprised? Didn't your grandmother put plaster of Paris in her bread? Didn't she dump sodium stearoyl-2-lactylate in the baking pan? Don't you remember the acrid aroma of azodicarbonamide wafting through her old-time kitchen? No? Hmmm, wonder how she got by. Anyway, plaster of Paris is nothing more than a chemical called calcium sulfate. It's great for patching cracks in the wall or for making it easier to knead 500-pound batches of dough in giant machines. Is it good for your tummy? Stop asking silly questions. Of course it isn't good for your tummy—but it makes better imitation bread. There are plenty of things that aren't good for you in imitation bread.

For example?

Well, for example, carrageenin is an extract of Irish moss—used as a thickener and dough conditioner. Recently the FDA put it on a special emergency list to be studied as a possible cause of cancer, birth defects, and other less-than-desirable effects.* But you can still get it in your bread. The FDA is supposed to be finished with the study in seven years, so until then just hang on.

Then there's propylene glycol. That's in your breakfast toast to keep it from becoming discolored while it lies on the supermarket shelf waiting for you to pick it up and take it home. Propylene glycol has another use too—it's better known as antifreeze. It doesn't cause much harm in animals, except it makes them awfully depressed. Been feeling depressed lately?

Diacetyl tartaric acid is an emulsifier used to save on shortening. It has never been adequately tested, and like all the rest of the junk on the list it has no place in bread. It is there for the convenience of the manufacturer and for no other reason.

But doesn't it keep the price of bread down?

When did you last notice the price of bread going down? When the big bakers insist that the chemicals in your daily loaf of cotton keep the price down, they mean it keeps the price down for *them,* not you. If you bought your whole wheat flour, salt, and yeast in large quantities you'd see how much cheaper real bread is than the imitation stuff.

And there's another problem with imitation bread— even the so-called 100 percent whole wheat bread that you

---

* *Gastroenterology*, 59:760, 1970.

buy at the supermarket has something wrong with it. It just isn't the same as the whole wheat bread you make at home. One reason is that all those creepy chemicals that get into white imitation bread also get into whole wheat imitation bread. The other problem is called "batter-whipping." It's a trick that the ice cream manufacturers have been using for years and the bread boys have recently caught on to. In making commercial ice cream, air is whipped into the final mix so that you are buying half ice cream and half air. That's why your ice cream is so soft and creamy. (The so-called hand-packed ice cream is much denser and much more expensive—it doesn't have all that air whipped into it.)

Supermarket bread, whether it's white, whole wheat, cinnamon raisin, oatmeal, or any other hokey variation on the theme, is whipped up with immense amounts of air to make that chemical-laden, shriveled little loaf look like real bread. Among themselves, bakers refer to the standard grocery store bread product as "balloon bread," and that's what it is. If it had just a little more air in it, it would fly right on up to the ceiling.

But what about other baked goods? Aren't they better than bread?

As long as they are made from "enriched" white flour, they can't be. The same rotten flour gets into pancakes, cake mixes, spaghetti, macaroni, waffles, home-baked pastry, pies, cookies, donuts, sweet rolls, crackers, hot dog and hamburger buns, turnovers, brownies, pizza dough, biscuits, breakfast squares, and every other flour or pasta product. If the raw material—the flour—has no nutrition, the final product can only be worse.

But if all those flour products aren't any good, how about breakfast cereals?

Brace yourself. There is no category of food product on the market that is more expensive, more profitable, and more nutritionally disastrous than breakfast cereals. To get a rapid understanding of exactly what the cereal companies are doing to us and to our children, let's take a hard look at one of the *better-quality* products on the market. A recent full-page ad for the cereal is a good place to start. The headline says: "WE DIDN'T MAKE BLANK BLANK CEREAL JUST FOR FUN."

Of course not. You made it for profit. Let's move over to the side of the package where all the action is:

"This delicious cereal is fortified with 8 important vitamins and 2 minerals."

Wait a minute. If it's such good stuff, why is it so lacking in nutrition that they have to fortify it with cheap synthetic vitamins and minerals sprayed on from a big spray gun at a cost of about one fourth of a cent? A fast look at the ingredients will give us the answer:

"Ingredients: sugar, corn, wheat, and oat flour, hydrogenated vegetable oil, salt, artificial coloring, sodium ascorbate, vitamin A palmitate, niacinamide, ascorbic acid, zinc oxide, iron, natural orange, lemon, cherry and other natural flavorings, thiamine hydrochloride, pyridoxine hydrochloride, riboflavin, folic acid, and vitamin D_2. BHA and BHT added to preserve product freshness."

Does that sound good? It shouldn't. The Food and Drug Administration requires that the ingredients be listed in order of quantity—that is, what there is most of has to go first and what there is least of has to appear last. So, according to the manufacturers, the largest single ingredient in this "cereal" is nothing but *cheap white refined sugar*.

How much sugar is there in the cereal?

Well, if you look down at the bottom of the side panel, you just might come across a little section entitled "carbohydrate information." If you majored in algebra and calculus, you should be able to calculate the sugar content from the figures given there: "sucrose and other sugars: 14 grams per 1 ounce." (If you think the combination of ounces and grams might be there to make the calculations harder for you, you just have a suspicious mind, that's all.)

Okay, here's the arithmetic:

There are 28.35 grams in one ounce so

$$\frac{14 \text{ grams}}{28.35 \text{ grams}} = 49.38\% \text{ sugar}$$

Pretty neat! Just by a whisker they missed selling you more sugar than cereal! But that's not all. There's another calculation we should do while we have the calculator out. In the same little corner of the box it says: "starch and related carbohydrates: 11 gm per ounce."

Applying the same formula

$$\frac{11 \text{ grams}}{28.35 \text{ grams}} = 38.8\% \text{ starch and related carbohydrates}$$

Hold on a minute! That means the breakfast "cereal" that you feed your kids to make them grow up healthy is *88.18 percent refined sugar and refined starch!* But do they really tell you to feed that product to your kids? Let's go back to the ad. It starts:

"If you have somebody under 12 years old in your house . . ." It goes on, ". . . they're different colors, they're ready sweetened, and they're about as much fun to eat as a cereal can be."

Eighty-eight point one eight percent refined sugar and refined starch and artificially colored makes them "fun to eat"?

But let's keep reading the ad:

"But that's just for kids' palates and funny bones. For their growing bodies, Blank Blank has a nutritional blend of corn, wheat, and oats . . ."

Do you believe that? Well, apparently the cereal manufacturer doesn't believe it either, because that's not what he says on the label. Let's take a look: "corn, wheat, and oat flour." That's not the same as "a nutritional blend of corn, wheat, and oats," is it? And there's a fascinating grammatical puzzle in that sentence. Does "corn, wheat, and oat flour" mean "corn and wheat in their natural form and oat flour" or does it mean "corn flour, wheat flour, and oat flour," or does it mean "corn plus wheat flour and oat flour"? Who knows? But any way you read it, it's not a "blend of corn, wheat, and oats," like they say in the ad. "Oat flour" has nothing like the nutritional value of real oats, and wheat flour is almost certainly the "enriched white flour" that we know so well.

But if they don't tell you the truth about that, will they tell you the truth about anything? Well, let's keep that in mind as we move on to the next ingredient.

That ingredient is "hydrogenated vegetable oil." Now you get an idea of how to make your own breakfast cereal. Take a cup of white refined sugar, add cornstarch, white wheat flour, and oat flour. Mix in a big slug of hydrogenated shortening—the stark white stuff like face cream they sell for baking—and mush it all together. Then roll it out in funny little shapes and bake it. Oh, yes, don't forget the chemicals and artificial coloring. Then set it out for your kids. But remember, don't let the dog have any of it. It might make him sick.

But what kind of vegetable oil do they use?

You can be sure it isn't $12-a-gallon imported Spanish olive oil. It might be the cheap yucky hydrogenated coconut oil that we've heard so much about already. But with all that sugar, you wouldn't notice another bad taste anyhow.

Next on the list of ingredients is "salt." It doesn't say exactly *how* much salt, but typically breakfast cereals for kids contain about 250 milligrams of salt per ounce, or about ten times as much as tiny little kiddy kidneys should be zapped with. But a lot of sugar and salt make the product ". . . about as much fun to eat as a cereal can be." Who cares about high blood presure and kidney damage from excessive salt during childhood?*

Next on the list is "artificial coloring." Your guess is as good as mine as to what that refers to. Let's just hope it isn't one of those notorious "U.S. Certified Pure Food Colors" that might be unmasked as a cause of cancer next week. And by the way, what's the purpose behind putting artificial colors in a product that *isn't* made "just for fun"?

---

* *Merck Manual of Diagnosis and Treatment.* Rahway, N.J., Merck & Co., 1972, p. 465.

Is the coloring there to sucker 4-year-olds into begging for it?

There's one more terrifying little detail that we shouldn't overlook. Remember that according to law the ingredients must be listed on the label in descending order of concentration? That means that this little box of "cereal" contains *more artificial coloring than vitamins!* The manufacturer makes a big deal of the fact that one ounce of their "cereal" gives you 25 percent of the Recommended Daily Allowance of some cheap and common vitamins. Wouldn't it be exciting if it also provided 10,000 percent of the Recommended Daily Allowance of artificial coloring?

But aren't those vitamins good for you?

If you want to buy cheap synthetic vitamins at a big price, then you'll be happy with this "cereal." But there's a clue to what you're getting right there on the label. You can get an idea of how nutritious a product is by checking the amount of nutrients it contains that weren't added artificially. In this case it's the magnesium, copper, phosphorus, and vital protein. You can get your full Recommended Daily Allowance of each of these important nutrients by choking down a mere three pounds of this "cereal" every day! Ugh!

Let's move fearfully to the final line in the list of ingredients: "BHA and BHT added to preserve product freshness."

Why do you say "fearfully"?

Because that's the right word. Those innocent little initials stand for the following fearsome chemical compounds:

BHA: butylated hydroxyanisole
BHT: butylated hydroxytoluene

Is that really what you want your kids to eat in their crunchy breakfast "cereal"? No, not when you hear what they really are.

BHA and BHT are chemical preservatives which have no place in your diet—much less the diet of your children. Their only purpose is to prevent the junky hydrogenated vegetable oil in the "cereal" from going rancid. A lot of food processors don't use any BHA/BHT at all—maybe they keep their plants cleaner than the competition, who knows? But what we do know is that the level of BHA/BHT can be as high as 0.1 percent in some foods. That's an interesting percentage because it corresponds exactly to the level in the food that rats were fed in a study in Australia. The rats didn't have too much trouble—just that their hair fell out and their blood cholesterol went through the roof. Of course, the baby rats born to rats who ate the same amount of BHA/BHT proportionately that you're probably eating did have some problems. They were born *without eyes*. Subsequent studies done at Loyola University in the United States confirmed this type of finding.*

Finally the FDA has gotten around to asking the companies who dope your food with BHA/BHT to please start animal tests to see if maybe these chemicals will make your wife give birth to a baby without eyes too. Doesn't it sound a little strange that the FDA is asking the companies to test their own product and then tell us if it's really safe? It's like the police putting an ad in the newspaper asking all criminals to report to the police station as soon as they commit a crime. Do you think the gigantic food processors are going to spend millions of dollars to discover that their profitable products are dangerous to you? Twenty years after everyone was convinced that cigarettes cause lung cancer, the cigarette companies are still insisting that cigarettes are safe and healthful.

In Britain they're a little smarter. The use of BHT in foods is forbidden—period. You don't need BHA/BHT; they can't make you healthy, and they can possibly make

---

* Winter, R., *Consumer's Dictionary of Food Additives*. New York, Crown Publishers, 1972. Jacobson, M., *Eater's Digest*. New York, Doubleday, 1972. FAO (31–41, 45); FAO (40A–28).

you sick. Don't buy or eat anything that contains them. If you still insist on buying breakfast "cereal," don't buy the kind that says: "BHA and BHT added to preserve product freshness."

Why do you always put the word "cereal" in quotation marks when you refer to breakfast cereal?

Because breakfast "cereal" isn't cereal. Cereal refers to a category of foods named after Ceres, the Roman goddess of grains. Cereals are things like wheat, barley, corn, oats, rye, rice, and the rest. Rice *flour* mixed with a lot of white sugar and hydrogenated coconut oil rolled into balls and baked in an oven is not a cereal. Oatmeal cooked in water and eaten hot is a cereal. If you don't like oatmeal, that's fine with me. (I don't like it either.) If you prefer cold cereal, try homemade granola as described in the *Save-Your-Life-High-Fiber Cookbook*. But let's not pretend that all the garbage in those seductive boxes on the grocery shelves is *real* cereal.

So there you have it. Breakfast "cereal" is a fascinating product: refined sugar and refined flour mixed with hydrogenated oil and salt. It contains more artificial coloring than vitamins, is almost 90 percent starch and sugar and preserved with chemicals that poison test animals. And the manufacturer takes out full-page ads that say: "'You'd be right as rain if you told your kids, 'Eat 'em! They're good for you!'" My friends, if you believe in a Day of Judgment, think twice before you give that advice to your children.

But if carbohydrates we eat are so bad and yet carbohydrates are so essential, how do we get *good* carbohydrates?

It isn't easy. Overrefined white flour is the basic raw material for most of the carbohydrate that Americans eat. If the flour is rotten, everything made with that flour is rotten. And the flour certainly is rotten—i.e., stripped of minerals, vitamins, and fiber. White flour and products made from it will make you fat, but worse than that, they can actually give you malnutrition—even on 3000 calories a day.

How can you get malnutrition on 3000 calories a day?

By eating overrefined carbohydrate. If 50 percent of your diet is lacking in vitamins, minerals, and fiber, you have to get 100 percent of your vitamins, minerals, and fiber from the other 50 percent of your diet. If you eat boxed breakfast "cereal," white "bread," white rice, and all the rest of the typical U.S. diet, you are depriving yourself of an important source of nutrition and starving your body of the elements it needs most. You will also—like 60 percent of all Americans—make yourself fat.

But don't all carbohydrates makes you fat?

That's what they'd like you to believe. But that little bit of nutritional fiction goes against *"The Nutritional Bill of Rights,"* which authoritatively states: *"All calories are created equal."* That means a calorie from beans has the same "fattening power" as a calorie from refined white sugar or wormlike white spaghetti or mushy white "bread." The catch is that you can eat a lot more slimy spaghetti than hard-to-chew beans.

A three-ounce serving of spaghetti contains a bare one tenth of a milligram of fiber—very little. The same size serving of white beans—the kind you eat in "pork and beans"—gives you 150 percent more fiber. You can get very fat on spaghetti and *you can't get fat on beans*.

Why is that?

It's the fiber that does it. Every unrefined carbohydrate also contains a good dose of fiber, and it's the fiber that keeps the carbohydrate honest. The fiber makes the food harder to chew and gets your jaws tired. The fiber soaks up water in your stomach, swells, and makes you feel stuffed. The fiber also cuts down the absorption of calories in the small intestine and lets you eat more without getting fat. But refining takes out the fiber and plies you with mushy, pasty, easy-to-gobble pap that doesn't fill you up.

Try the comparison of an apple and a slice of white "bread." Both of them supply about 60 calories—the apple has plenty of fiber, the white "bread" almost none. If you're having a little lunch, you can easily down four skimpy pasty little slices of white "bread." But one apple is about all the average person can eat—but let's say two apples just to make it extra fair. Two apples: 120 calories. Four slices of white bread: 240 calories. Just go through the average day doubling your caloric intake and see how long it takes you to start buying tent dresses and nice baggy pants.

Does that apply to all the foods made with refined carbohydrate?

It sure does. A cookie made with whole wheat flour is filling and nourishing; a white-flour cookie is oversweetened mush. Haven't you noticed how your kids can eat a dozen at a time? A slice of high-fiber cake fills you up; a slice of low-fiber cake fattens you up. It's even worse with fruits. One cup of fresh raw pineapple gives you 73 calories. One cup of unsweetened canned pineapple *juice* gives you 138 calories—again almost double. And it takes a lot more pineapple juice to fill you up than slices of *fresh* pineapple. An orange checks in at 88 calories, but a bottle of orange pop comes through at 160 calories. The orange is loaded with nutrients and fiber; the pop is loaded with gas and calories—period.

But why do food manufacturers insist on making their products with refined white flour instead of natural whole wheat flour?

Because they are in the business of selling cookies or pizzas—not in the business of selling better health. There are a lot of insignificant reasons to use white flour in mass-produced garbage foods like snack crack crackers, breakfast brownies, frozen waffles and white "bread." White flour is easier to mix, stores longer, it has greater "consumer acceptability" because we've been educated to believe that white is "clean" and everyone wants to be "clean," and it's smooth—all Americans like things that are smooth. But the biggest incentive for manufacturers to use millions of tons of worthless white flour in your food and your children's food is that they make more money that way. It's just a matter of fiber.

What difference does the fiber make?

Suppose you're in the food business and you sell real whole wheat bread at the same price as awful cottony white "bread." The high-fiber content of the whole wheat bread fills up the customers fast and they eat much less—at least 50 percent less. That means you sell only half as much bread and make half the profit. That means a smaller yacht, a Cadillac Seville instead of the DeVille, and a house in the unfashionable part of Beverly Hills. The same scientific principle applies to cookies, cakes, pretzels, pies, and cakes. It also covers cake mixes, pancake mixes, biscuit mixes, and every other kind of flour-based mix. The average housewife buys nearly two boxes of cake mix a week. Give her a high-fiber mix and she'd only need one, because her family would be satisfied with one cake a week. They would also lose weight, feel better, and live longer. But the entire food-processing industry is based on the concept of selling you expensive low-fiber, high-sugar, and high-salt foods that *don't fill you up*—so as soon as you finish one cupcake you'll be right back in line for another one.

And the food processors spend billions of dollars a year telling you how "good" products made with overrefined carbohydrates are. General Foods, for example, in 1973 spent a mere $180 million in advertising. The other "General," General Mills, signed checks for almost $75 million to advertise their products the same year. The 28 biggest advertisers in the food business spent about $2 billion to sell their basically low-fiber, overrefined carbohydrate products. The only group in the country that has the same kind of financial clout is the U.S. government, and in that year their budget to promote high-fiber unrefined carbohydrates was exactly: *nothing.* So the score stands—Refined Carbohydrates: $2 billion, Natural Carbohydrates: zero. This year won't be any better.

What's the solution?

One solution is a "Carbohydrate Survival Plan" for you and your family. It will lower your food costs by at least 30 percent—and maybe as much as 50 percent. It will cut down—or eliminate—tooth decay and dental bills. It will solve the problem of obesity once and for all. It will give you substantial protection against diabetes, heart attacks, diverticulosis, and cancer of the colon. And last, but far from least, it will provide you with a better tasting, more satisfying diet. This is the way it works:

Just make up two food lists, a YES list and a NO list. Don't eat anything on the NO list if you can possibly avoid it, and do your best to eat only foods on the YES list. That's all. Here are the lists:

NO

1. Any product containing refined sugar: that includes corn syrup, sucrose, dextrose, lactose, corn sugar, or any of the other aliases for refined sugar.
2. Any product containing refined flour: that means don't

140

eat any flour product unless it states precisely: "100% whole wheat," "100% whole rye," "100% whole oat," and the like—*and no other flour content*.

3. Don't eat processed fruits or vegetables. That means eat nothing that comes in cans, jars, bottles, frozen in boxes, dehydrated, or otherwise mutilated.

4. Avoid all soft drinks except those you make yourself at home. (See YES list for details.)

5. Avoid all bottled and canned sauces, such as ketchup, salad dressing, steak sauce, and barbecue sauce, from the supermarket. These concoctions contain massive amounts of refined carbohydrates in the form of white flour and refined sugar.

6. Avoid most pre-prepared "snack foods" such as crackers, "cheese nibblies," crispy onion-flavored "yum-yums," and all the other moronic names. They are a massive source of the refined carbohydrate that will help to damage your health, sex appeal, and bank account.

What about the YES list?

Here it comes:

1. Consume only unrefined sweeteners and products containing unrefined sweeteners. That means use honey, unrefined molasses, pure maple syrup, and unrefined sugar.

2. Use only foods from or containing 100 percent whole grain cereals without refined sugar. That eliminates at one fell swoop all boxed breakfast cereals, since even those that contain bran or whole wheat are liberally dosed with sugar. For example, a popular bran "cereal" is a whopping 6 percent sugar by weight.

Good-bye to pies, cakes, cookies, instant pizzas, and all the rest of commercial flour-based products. Also forget about the supermarket so-called whole wheat bread, and the exotic mixtures of flours that have exciting little stories about the people in other countries who conquered the world by eating them. Just check the list of ingredients—if you can find it on the many-colored wrapper—and you'll see the number-one ingredient is usually "flour" or "wheat flour." That doesn't mean *"whole* wheat flour," my friend.

3. Eat only fresh fruits and vegetables as nearly in their original form as possible. That means potatoes in their skins, apples with the peel (and the core and the seeds if you feel like it), brown rice, fresh melons, and so on.

4. Make your own soft drinks using natural sweeteners and natural fruits. You can make an orange drink with oranges and water—in the blender if you like—that your kids can drink all day without getting fat and sick. It won't rot your teeth either. Don't worry about diluting the orange juice—commercial orange drinks contain as little as 10 percent real orange substance anyway. (The most expensive orange beverage, orange soda pop, contains hardly any real orange at all.) You can do the same with pineapple, apple, pear, banana, strawberry, lemon, lime, coconut, and dozens of others.

5. Make your own condiments—they will be better tasting, cheaper, and much more fun. Salad dressing is oil and vinegar with spices; prepared mustard is ground mustard seed with water and sweetener. Ketchup is tomatoes with vinegar and sweetener; most commercial ketchup is half-rotten tomatoes and tons of cheapie corn sugar. You can make a better product with your eyes closed.

6. Instead of food-factory "snack foods," eat real-world snack foods. Try nuts, seeds, popcorn, whole-grain crackers, sesame seed cookies, peanut-butter balls rolled in coconut, and the thousand other possibilities. In the same way you can make your own pies, cakes, cookies, pizza, and even spaghetti and noodles. (Just add water, salt, and eggs to whole wheat flour, roll it around a little bit and crank it through a $25 pasta machine. You'll have instant high-fiber pasta or noodles and your savings will pay for your machine before you know it.)

But if I follow those lists, won't I be paying a lot more instead of a lot less for my food?

Nope. Your food costs will go down. But what if your food costs went up because you ate a better diet? Would it be worth it? Isn't it better to spend the money at the food store instead of the doctor's office and the drugstore? Is there a better investment that anyone can make than the construction and maintenance of their own body? Is it smart to eat poor-quality food and buy a good-quality car?

But you don't even have to contemplate those questions. Good, natural, wholesome food is cheaper than junk. If the average American family just eliminated soda pop from their diet, they would cut their food costs at least 10 percent—and maybe more. How many cans of pop at 25 or more cents a can does your family consume a week? How many expensive jars of powdered imitation orange juice and how many big cans of high-cost imitation fruit punches do they guzzle a week? Just add it up. How much do you spend on bottled salad dressing and barbecue sauce every month? How many hard-earned dollars go down the drain in your house for junky cookies, awful snack crackers, worthless breakfast "cereals"?

But hasn't it been proved by the United States Department of Agriculture in official tests that convenience foods cost less than making them yourself from scratch?

If you believe *that*, you'll believe *anything*. In a comparison that must have warmed the hearts of the food-processing industry, the USDA compared the prices of preparing certain food items from scratch with buying the "same" foods already prepared. The only trouble is that they weren't the "same" foods at all.

What do you mean, they weren't the "same"?

Take chow mein, for example. The USDA used two different recipes to make the comparison. The canned super-

143

market chow mein recipe had a big ½ ounce of chicken. The homemade version called for 2⅓ ounces of chicken. Guess which one the USDA said was cheaper? Right— canned chow mein. But if the amount of chicken is made equal—the only fair way—the canned chow mein is at least 460 percent more expensive. They played the same dummy game with frozen pork-fried rice. The supermarket version contained the usual ½ ounce of pork, but the USDA insisted that what you make at home has to have 2⅓ ounces. Back when I went to school, we used to call this "cheating." Now I guess it's known as "marketing."

The USDA seems to be telling us that the best way to lower your food costs is to pay high prices for cans of inferior factory-made food with microscopic amounts of meat and chicken. Why do they do that?

Is there anything else to know about the "Carbohydrate Survival Plan"?

That's about it. Strangely enough, it works out to be about the same as the high-fiber diet I've written about previously. Actually it's two ways of arriving at the same desirable goal. I can make one fascinating guarantee: If you try the "Carbohydrate Survival Plan" completely for one month, you'll never want to go back to your old way of eating. In addition, you will reduce your food bill in ways that you never before imagined.

That sounds fine, but didn't you leave out the most dangerous carbohydrate of all, table sugar?

Nope. Just see Chapter X.

CHAPTER IX
Protein

_____

Why do we hear so much about how important it is to eat a lot of protein?

Because there's a lot of profit in protein. Protein has become a status food, a political football, a pseudoscientific fad, and a high-profit supermarket seller all at the same time. The truth is: *there is no magic in protein.* You need relatively small amounts in your diet, and it's easy to get it if you know where to look for it. You can find cheap sources of protein that taste better, provide better nutrition, and will help you live longer than a fatty slab of beefsteak. But to do that you have to know what protein really is.

What is protein, really?

Protein is nothing more or less than a collection of common chemical substances called *amino acids*. These amino acids are hooked together like pearls on a string to form protein. There are about twenty-two amino acids that combine to form almost all the proteins known to man. Of these twenty-two, eight (more or less*) are called

_____

* "More or less" is about as close as nutritionists get to agreeing on amino acids. There are a couple of others that *might* be "essential" for children, but 8 is the usual figure given for the basic "essentials" for adults.

essential amino acids. These are the amino acids that the body is not *supposed* to be able to manufacture itself. The cycle of proteins and amino acids in the body consists of three simple steps:

1. You eat a protein food.
2. Your body digests the protein—breaking it down into its component amino acids. In a sense, it's like taking the pearls in a necklace off the string.
3. Your body then reassembles the amino acid "pearls" to form new patterns of protein that your body can use.

Every protein-eating animal does the same thing, although the patterns of protein are different for each species. For example, when a cat eats a mouse, its digestive system disassembles the proteins of the mouse tissues, breaks them down into amino acids, and reassembles those amino acids into cat protein.

What are the essential amino acids?

These are their names, although we will see that they aren't nearly as "essential" as we have been led to believe: lysine, methionine, leucine, threonine, valine, tryptophan, isoleucine, and phenylalanine. (There are two others sometimes considered essential for kids: arginine and histidine.)

It has long been a textbook principle of "nutrition" that if a protein food does *not* contain all of these eight essential amino acids in sufficient amounts, it loses some of its value as a source of protein to the body. Nobody disagrees with that statement. But—and it's a big BUT—professional nutritionists, especially those on the payroll of the giant food processors, have gone one step farther. They tell us, in newspaper articles and textbooks, that "no protein can be considered worthwhile unless it contains all the essential amino acids in just the right proportion."

According to *them*, only three categories of food qualify as complete protein: eggs, milk products, and animal flesh. If that were true—*and it isn't*—it would be good news for meat packers, dairy farmers, and egg sellers. It would also mean the end of the human race, since about two billion residents of this planet get little if any of those foods. Apparently the residents of less fortunate nations than the United States know something that our professors of nutrition don't know.

What do they know?

They know that ten dimes are just as good as a one-dollar bill—maybe better. If you can't afford a pound of porterhouse steak, with its eight essential amino acids, why not just settle for a dish of brown rice? The rice will give you about 5 grams of protein, but unfortunately that protein will be deficient in two essential amino acids: isoleucine and lysine. That means your body won't really get the most benefit from the protein in the rice. Okay, how about eating a nice dish of black beans instead? A steaming bowl of black beans will give you about 12 grams of protein. But there's a catch: the black beans have plenty of isoleucine and lysine, but they are short of some of the sulfur-containing essential amino acids. Do you have to rush out to the supermarket for three-dollar-a-pound, not-so-tender beefsteak just to keep alive? I don't think so. Just pour the beans on top of the rice and mix them around. The beans provide the amino acids that the rice lacks, and the rice adds the missing amino acids to the beans. Suddenly you have a "complete" and perfect protein. The cost is about twenty-two cents instead of three dollars, and there are plenty of other advantages that we will see in the next few pages.

This is a good time to take a look at the place of meat as a source of protein in a good diet.

Then meat is an excellent source of protein?

Nope. It's an excellent source of surprises—most of them unpleasant. How about a fast true-or-false quiz? Okay? Here goes:

1. The only way to get all the essential amino acids is to eat meat.
2. Meat contains more protein than other foods.
3. You must have meat in your diet to assure an adequate protein intake.
4. There are some essential vitamins and minerals you can only get from meat.
5. People who eat a lot of meat are better fed than those who don't.
6. Meat gives you the best *quality* protein available.

I know. When I went to grade school the teacher used to roll out those nice big colored charts and tell all us little kids the Gospel about Good Red Meat. She said, bless her heart, that all six statements above were the absolute truth. She was *wrong*. And if we still believe what she said, we are *wrong*. And the meat sellers who still insist that it's all true—they are doubly *wrong* because *they know better*.

Here are the correct answers:

1. Nope. You can get all the essential amino acids—as well as the nonessential ones—better and cheaper from eggs, milk, or vegetables.
2. Certainly not. Any way you look at it, there are other foods that contain more protein than meat—certain cheeses, for one example.
3. Not at all. There are more than three quarters of a *billion* vegetarians on this planet, including the Hindus of India, the Seventh-Day Adventists worldwide, and others. They are notably healthier than other similar populations who consume large amounts of meat.
4. Hardly. Nutritionally there is nothing special about meat except its tendency to spoil almost instantly without refrigeration. Every essential element can be found better and cheaper in other foods.
5. Regrettably false. A lot of meat in the diet fills you up too fast and displaces fresh fruits, vegetables, fiber, and cereals from your diet. Because of its high fat content, meat can also make you fat fast.
6. Sorry. The best quality protein by far resides in those

little cackleberries called eggs. Compared with the fruit of the noble hen, meat is in far left field.

But that goes against everything we've been taught. Are you sure it's true?

Sure I'm sure. I know it's just as shocking to you as it was to me, but once we understand the rules of the protein game, it all comes into focus. There are only two basic things to remember:

1. Protein *quantity*.
2. Protein *quality*.

Let's take protein *quantity* first. It's an easy calculation to make. Obviously a nice lamb chop contains much more protein than a serving of beans, doesn't it? *No, it doesn't.* A raw lamb chop is 14.7 percent protein, while raw soybeans are 34.1 percent protein. Parmesan cheese is 36 percent protein, and even cheapie American cheese is 25 percent protein. It's hard to find any kind of meat that checks in at more than 30 percent protein. Cow's milk is only 3.5 percent protein at best, although dry skim milk can be as much as 36 percent protein—which opens up another way to pick your pocket, but more about that later on. In calculating the "value" of protein-containing foods, the actual percentage of protein in that food is a useful consideration.

But *quantity* of protein is no big deal. Much more important is how efficiently your body can use all those expensive proteins you are pouring into it. Unless you know the rules of the protein game you—and your children—will end up *overfed* and *undernourished*.

That brings us to the second point—*quality* of protein. In this case "quality" has nothing to do with the number of transistors in a stereo or whose name is on the label of a pair of twenty-five-dollar jeans. In the world of protein, "quality" means pedigree—how many and how much of the eight essential amino acids each kind of protein brings to your body. The string of amino acids that make up a protein may have as little as 51 amino acids or as many as 200,000, but that's beside the point. The only thing you have to ask about protein quality is: "Are those eight essential amino acids there, and is there enough of each one?"

How much is "enough" amino acid?

A good question. The human digestive system has a hard time storing amino acids. Once a protein food is digested and disassembled into its various amino acids, they must be used promptly. Any amino acids that are not immediately utilized in the body metabolism are immediately converted into fat or carbohydrate. (That's one of the reasons why a high-protein diet can make you into a butterball faster than you think.) So, the way it works out is, a protein is only as good as its amino acids. It's something like a club meeting with eight officers—unless all of them are there, there's no quorum and nothing gets accomplished. Unless all the essential amino acids are present and unless there is enough of each one, the *quality* of the protein is diminished. If a protein food has 100 percent of your requirements of seven of the essential amino acids and only 50 percent of your requirements of the eighth essential amino acid, it is considered to be only half as good as a protein that contains all eight essential amino acids in full strength.

Then you should only eat protein that has all the essential amino acids in full strength?

That's what they'd like you to believe. For the past forty years that's been the "Official Nutrition Doctrine," and it's been very effective in selling massive amounts of fatty meat to frightened housewives who try to save their already overweight families from protein "deficiency." In reality, the whole mythology about protein is a combination of superstition and nutritional blackmail. That's what the textbooks on nutrition say, that's what they teach the kids in school (that's what they taught you and me), and not by accident, that's what the major food processors drum into our brains constantly. It's a great way to force massive amounts of overpriced meat, cheese, eggs, and milk down our unsuspecting throats. But nutritionally and scientifically it just doesn't make any sense.

But what makes you think that you know better than all the experts in nutrition?

Because there are no "experts" in nutrition. In the world of science we all have access to the same facts, and if we consider those facts honestly, we almost have to arrive at the same conclusions. However, if we were to receive $40,000 a year in grants from a gigantic company that peddles breakfast food or from a meat-packers trade association, then we just might develop a little blind spot insofar as the nutritional values of our benefactor's products are concerned. But by the time you finish this book, you will be able to cut through all the half-truths and distortions that the food companies have unleashed on you and stand up to any alleged nutritionist who tells you that awful white sugar is good for you or that boxed breakfast cereal is a decent food for your children. A good place to start is with the peddlers of protein. Let's go back to the mythology of amino acids.

What about the mythology of amino acids?

Just this. You don't have to eat a food that has all eight essential amino acids in perfect proportions to get your protein requirements. All you have to do is eat one food that has some of the essential amino acids at about the same time you eat another food that has the rest of the essential amino acids. That's all.

And guess what? That's what the human race has been doing since it began. Whole wheat bread is deficient in one of the essential amino acids, *lysine*. Cheese has plenty of lysine. So people have been eating a lot of bread with a little cheese on it for thousands of years. In the Caribbean, the natives eat rice and peas. The rice is short of isoleucine and lysine (as we noticed previously), and the peas are short of tryptophan. But together, they have all the essential amino acids in the quantities required. In India they eat wheat and lentils or peas or beans. In Latin America the favorite dish is rice and black beans, or as they call it, "Christians and Moros." All these dishes and dozens of others like them provide people with all the essential amino acids they need. If humans couldn't get their total protein requirement from simple, inexpensive nonmeat foods, the race would have died out long ago.

But how much of these essential amino acids does a person need?

Much less than you would think from reading all the scare articles about protein "deficiency." If only one fifth of all the protein you eat in a day is made up of essential amino acids, you will be in excellent shape.* That means if you eat three ounces of good protein a day (much more than sufficient, as we will shortly see), all you need to satisfy your essential amino acid requirements is a little over a half ounce of protein containing that magic combination of the eight essential amino acids. *In reality it's almost impossible for any normal person to avoid getting more than enough protein each and every day.* That's the real reason why protein deficiency is virtually unknown in the United States or any major industrialized country—except among people who are sick with other serious diseases where eating a ton of protein a day wouldn't help them. And—get ready for this—it seems that even those sacred eight essential amino acids aren't so sacred or so essential.

How can that be?

Well, see what the famous National Academy of Sci-

---

* National Academy of Sciences, *Recommended Dietary Allowances*, 8th ed. Washington, D.C., 1974, p. 44.

ences has to say: "Since cystine can replace part of the requirement for methionine, and tyrosine part of that for phenylalanine, these too must be considered in evaluating diets."* That means that cystine and tyrosine—both manufactured within your body and not essential amino acids—can substitute for part of at least two of the *essential* amino acids.

So you need far less of those eight amino acids than you have been led to believe. As a matter of fact, you need far less protein than the food processors have been telling you.

How much protein do you actually need?

Probably not nearly as much as you are eating currently. Most people massively overconsume protein under the delusion that in some magical way it will make them strong.

To actually calculate how much protein a person needs a day, we should know how much he uses up. In the human body, protein exists in a dynamic state—that is, the protein you eat is digested and broken down into amino acids. These amino acids are then assembled to make new proteins your body can use. As your own body tissues are used up, the amino acids that are thrown off are recycled into fresh protein. But there is an unavoidable daily loss of protein from urine, feces, sweat, and sloughed-off skin. Every time you cut yours nails or get a haircut you lose vital protein.

An average 150-pound man on an average day loses about 23 grams of protein—or a mere eight tenths of an ounce. So it would seem reasonable to expect a good diet to replace all the protein that is lost. That means an adult should get along fine on eight tenths of an ounce of protein a day, or about a pound and a half of protein per month. In technical terms, that's known as *nitrogen balance*—or *protein balance,* since protein is measured chemically in terms of nitrogen.

* National Academy of Sciences, *Recommended Dietary Allowances,* 8th ed. Washington, D.C., 1974, p. 44.

Even the National Academy of Sciences says: "In healthy individuals there is little evidence of nutritional benefit from intakes of protein that exceed requirements." Then they go on to recommend that the same 150-pound man consume *a massive 68 grams of protein a day,* or almost three times the amount that he needs to maintain perfect protein balance.

Where did you get your figures for protein requirements?

Wait. You haven't heard them yet. Reliable scientific organizations unanimously recommend about 32 grams of protein a day for the "average" 150-pound man—less for women. That's just a shade over an ounce of protein daily, or about half the standard textbook, newspaper column, and magazine article recommendation.

The sources for these figures are:

1. *Evaluation of Protein Nutrition,* NAS/NRC, Washington, D.C., Pamphlet #711.
2. *Canadian Bulletin on Nutrition,* Dietary Standard for Canada, 1964.
3. *Protein Requirements,* Food and Agricultural Organization, World Health Organization Expert Group, United Nations Conference, Rome, 1965.

But then these august bodies add on an "extra" requirement of a whopping *30 percent,* to bring the "requirement" to about 42 grams of protein a day.

Who needs that extra allowance of protein?

The people who sell meat, fish, cheese, eggs, chicken, and all the other high-prestige and expensive sources of protein. Raising the amount of protein you eat by 30 percent raises their incomes 30 percent. It also increases the amount of protein in the sewers and septic tanks of your neighborhood 30 percent as you merrily urinate away everything that you can't use that very day. It also deprives the starving children of the world of the protein that would save their lives. Incidentally it makes you pay 30 percent of your already bloated food bill for protein that you never will use. If you are an average American family, it will cost you about $40 a month to unnecessarily pump up your protein intake. That puts another *$36 billion* a year into the pockets of the protein producers.

And what do you get for that money? You get more protein products in your daily urine flow than the average African has in his daily diet. You decide if that's what you want.

But let's dig a little deeper into the scientific facts. Even the minimum allowance of 23 grams of protein a day to replace your normal protein losses may be too much. It turns out that if you eat less protein—within limits—your body uses that protein more efficiently. You waste less and you need less.

In scientific slang it goes: "First, subjects consuming a low-protein or protein-free diet undergo many types of adaptations (Waterlow, 1968) that tend to improve nitrogen (protein) conservation."*

Furthermore, the closer you get to fulfilling the small minimum protein requirements, the more protein you waste. Here it is in the stilted words of nutritional pig-Latin: "Observations on man indicate that high-quality proteins and the proteins of many mixed diets are utilized with only 65–70 percent efficiency when consumed in amounts approaching the requirements."† So about a third of that high-priced protein goes down the drain most of the time in the overproteined American diet.

But what about NPU?

I can see you've been doing your homework. NPU

* National Academy of Sciences, *Recommended Dietary Allowances*, 8th ed. Washington, D.C., 1974, p. 44.
† *Ibid.*, p. 46.

stands for "Net Protein Utilization" and is a nifty way to confuse the public. All protein foods are given a rating based on their protein *quantity* and the amount and varieties of amino acids they contain. A high NPU score is a wonderful thing in the minds of some nutritionists, and a low NPU is supposed to be something to be ashamed of. But God created low NPU proteins as well as high NPU products, and guess what? Generally speaking, the higher the NPU, the higher the price. Eggs, milk, fish, poultry, and cheese are right up there—both in NPU score and in pulling the plug on your already leaky checking account.

If you eat the usual variety of fresh foods every day, you can even forget what NPU stands for—it couldn't concern you less. And even if you don't eat a variety of fresh foods every day, you're almost sure to still get your protein allowance. Remember, all you need is something close to an ounce or so of protein every twenty-four hours.

Even the poor farmers in Latin America get their minimum protein allowances—if they eat the native foods—and they never heard of NPU or amino acids. For example, a few corn tortillas plus some beans with a tiny sliver of cheese once in a while and an occasional egg provide all the protein a hardworking farmer needs. (In a few pages we'll do all the magical nutritionists' calculations to prove it's true in theory as well as in practice.)

But doesn't someone who works hard need extra protein?

What for? Protein serves the function of replacing enzymes, rebuilding blood cells, producing antibodies, and replenishing mucus among other things. None of those elements are damaged by doing physical work. Let's check with the ultradistinguished National Academy of Sciences again: "There is little evidence that muscular activity increases the need for protein."*

Any protein you eat—beyond that approximate necessary ounce or so—will not make you stronger or happier or more attractive. It will not develop the breasts of wom-

* National Academy of Sciences, *Recommended Dietary Allowances*, 8th ed. Washington, D.C., 1974, p. 43.

en, increase the sexual potency of men, or make little children get better grades in school. These, and all the other claims made for protein, are designed to fortify the bank accounts of hustlers who peddle high-protein concentrates and other similar nostrums. Americans and other gullibles spend millions of dollars every month on "Super High Protein Cosmic Concentrate" or "Oriental Protein Essence" or "Power-Packed Protein Powder." Basically all this snake-oil product-identification boils down (and "boils down" is the right expression) to three primary mixtures. The only thing they have in common is that they are astronomically overpriced.

The first kind of high-protein supplement is *literally* boiled down from the hooves of pigs and the stomachs of cows swept up from the floor of the slaughterhouse. The sticky gooey substance that comes out of the big boiling pots has two uses: glue for furniture or "high-protein supplement" for the foolish. The glue runs about fifty cents a pound; a pound of "high-protein supplement" will set you back eight dollars. The protein content is the same, but don't eat the glue—they purposely make it dirty so you won't be tempted.

Another "high-protein" hustle is based on plain old powdered skim milk. It *is* high in protein and it does have a lot of amino acids—but it's certainly nothing out of this world. The protein peddlers dope it up with sugar, some fancy flavorings, and a list of amino acids so long that it looks like it's going to run off the page. But the plain old supermarket dry skim milk has the same amino acids, no sugar, and sells for about one tenth the price.

The third kind of "protein concentrate" is soybean flour. Most soy flour is not just ground-up soybeans—oh no, that would be too straightforward. Soybeans contain a valuable cooking oil used in many common brands. For example, Wesson Oil is a combination of soybean and cottonseed oil, Crisco Oil is soybean oil, as are some other national brands. There is nothing wrong with soy oil for cooking, but the economics are interesting. After the oil is pressed out of the beans, it is sold at wholesale for about twenty-two cents a pound. (That comes out to about eighty-five cents a quart for the unrefined oil.) The dry mash that is

left is known as soybean meal and is usually sold for animal feed.* The wholesale price is about $150 a ton or
seven and a half cents a pound. That's where your soybean flour probably comes from. It is high in protein but
deficient in at least one essential amino acid: methionine.
That doesn't mean much—unless you're paying eight dollars a pound for the wrung-out soybean meal as a "high-
protein supplement." There's also a whole new world of
food flim-flam that depends on the soybean.

What's that all about?

It's all about high prices for cheap ingredients, pious
pronouncements, and the usual thinly veiled death threats.
Food processors have always found the best way to sell a
product is to threaten their customers with death if they
don't use it. That's why people buy all that "polyunsaturated" (joke) margarine, oil, mayonnaise, shortening,
and the rest of the assorted fats. That's also why they take
vitamins and minerals and "protein supplements" and
drink millions of gallons more than they need of citrus
juices and milk.

The ads say subtle little things like: "To stay
healthy . . ." or "To keep in the peak of condition . . ." or,
more menacingly, "For the sake of your heart . . ." and
"Ask your doctor . . ." But behind every hard sell in the
food industry is the hint that the Angel of Death will bear
you swiftly away if you don't consume their product. As
we have seen, sometimes your best chance of living to collect your pension might be to do just the opposite of what
those $32,000 four-color full-page ads try to scare you into
doing.

Now back to soybeans. Recently a whole new "product
line" has appeared on the market using a powder known
as "textured vegetable protein" or TVP for short. It's made
of soy protein mixed with a haphazard collection of chemicals and molded to imitate common foods. It is used to

---

* Actually the defatted soybean meal has more protein per pound,
since there is no space taken up by the soybean oil that has been
squeezed out. But still, no magic.

"stretch" more expensive foods without significantly lowering their price. A good example is hamburger at the butcher shop which is sold at a slightly lower price mixed with up to 30 percent TVP. There are two problems—TVP isn't hamburger and the price doesn't get lowered that much. At least in the butcher shop they tell you (or they *should* tell you) that you're buying beef and getting soybeans. But in schools, hospitals, restaurants, and especially fast-food joints, TVP is like a dream-come-true. It's a cheapie ingredient that can be used to stretch expensive meat, and the customer can't taste it and you don't have to tell him. No wonder TVP is considered a big "profit-builder." Wow! And you can make it taste like sausage, chicken, pork, ham, nuts, or almost anything else. It can even come out looking and tasting *almost* like bacon. Want the recipe? Here it is:

Almost Bacon: TVP, yeast, soy protein, salt, artificial flavoring, monosodium glutamate, stabilizer, vegetable oil, artificial coloring, water

That's not bacon any way you look at it. But the next time you eat out, look at your salad. That stuff you thought was crumbled-up bits of cooked bacon may be your first conscious introduction to the new world of "almost" foods. Good appetite.

But aren't soybeans the perfect solution to the world shortage of protein?

What world shortage of protein? First of all, in the United States and most industrial nations, no one can even suggest that there is a shortage of protein. A much bigger worry is the strain on human kidneys from the massive amounts of protein they have to process in the urine every day. (Protein, you know, just doesn't trickle out of the body. It requires hard work on the part of both kidneys to get rid of all the excessive and unneeded protein Americans consume each day.)

Now let's take a look at the world protein situation.

Americans on the average consume over 90 grams of protein a day—about three times what they need. But New Zealanders and Yugoslavs eat more—over 100 grams a day in the case of New Zealand and slightly less for the Yugoslavs. Mexicans eat about 70 grams daily, and even the poorest eaters of all, the Central and West Africans, put away a hefty 55 grams of protein on the average per person per day. That's even more than it seems, since babies and old people and children and most women don't eat nearly that much, although they are counted in the averages. The average 150-pound man of the statistics who needs approximately an ounce (or 28 grams) of protein is eating 150 percent more than he needs. And that is in the poorest areas of the world.* Making allowances for the fact that some of the protein is of animal origin—although eating various grains together makes them just as good or better than meat and fish—such a diet still provides almost everyone with enough protein for adequate growth and development. So, folks, it's not time to start chomping soybeans yet—if you can avoid it, that is.

But can't we help these people anyway?

What about helping ourselves first? American children have, without any shadow of a doubt, the worst diet of any children in the world. A poor child of the Middle East eats coarse whole wheat bread, cheese, brown rice, camel or goat's milk, an occasional egg, and fresh fruits and vegetables. An affluent American child eats imitation white "bread," breakfast "cereal" coated with massive amounts of white sugar, and drinks imitation orange-flavored breakfast drink. His unsuspecting mother doses him with canned spaghetti and meat (?) balls, imitation potato chips, and frozen TV dinners. And the children in foreign countries need *us* to help *them*?

The few feeble attempts to supply proteins to foreign populations have been disasters. Just because a nation doesn't eat the same brands as we do or doesn't gobble

---

* Mayer, J., The dimensions of human hunger. *Scientific American,* Sept. 1976, p. 45.

everything out of cans doesn't mean they suffer from nutritional problems. For example, someone in Washington, D.C., once got the bright idea that black African tribesmen would eat better if we sent them some of our powdered skim milk. After all, it is a "high-protein" food (although not *that* high, as we have seen), and it would get rid of a big surplus of powdered milk that the Agriculture Department bought from farmers to keep the price you pay at the supermarket right up there. So governmental nutritional "experts" analyzed the diets of the Africans without paying much attention to the food combinations that they were eating in calculating protein intake. The "experts" concluded that the blacks weren't getting enough animal protein and selected them to receive a big shipment of slightly overage powdered skim milk.

What happened?

Just what you might have predicted. The very fact that the African tribes were still in existence after thousands of years of exposure to all the hazards of primitive living should have suggested that they didn't need our help in the food department. But there was one other factor that the Washington experts didn't think of.

Orientals and blacks are not the same genetically as whites. That's obvious. One of the important differences is a deficiency in their bodies of a chemical enzyme called *lactase.* Lactase is essential in the digestion of milk; if you give milk to a person who lacks lactase, he gets sick. He gets abdominal pains, nausea, vomiting, diarrhea, and all the rest. That's why milk is not a prominent item in the diets of most Japanese and Chinese and many blacks.

The Africans gratefully accepted the wonderful powdered skim milk from their American benefactors—they accepted tons of it, in fact. They mixed it with water and tried to drink it. They got sick. They tried to drink it again. They got sicker. They stopped drinking it. But they were poor people accustomed to making the best of a hard existence. The powdered skim milk that you pay for at the corner grocery did not go to waste.

What happened to it?

In that particular part of Africa, that particular tribe has the whitest mud huts of any tribe anywhere. Each day little black boys dip their brushes in fabulously expensive high-protein skim milk and carefully whitewash the brown mud walls of their family dwelling. And they really appreciate it. At least that's what I'm told.

What does a good protein diet consist of?

Good proteins. And good proteins have the following qualities:

1. They are relatively free of fat, so that your daily protein dose doesn't ruin your health in the process.
2. They are inexpensive, so that a decent diet doesn't ruin your bank account.
3. They are appetizing and satisfying, so you are motivated to eat them.

The typical American diet flops on almost every count. The primary source of protein for most Americans is gigantic globs of meat accompanied by low-fiber low-protein vegetables and an overdose of chemical-laden factory-made convenience foods. Most Americans also swig a lot of cow's milk—in one form or another—under the delusion that they are getting good expensive protein that way. They aren't. And there are a couple of good reasons for this massive misinformation about nutrition.

What reasons are those?

First are the so-called trade associations, which function as nutritional shock troops to frighten you into eating *their* favorite foods. On a national television program I once suggested that the proven cancer-causing chemical diethylstilbestrol, which is prohibited in sixty countries, didn't belong in the beef that you buy at the supermarket. One of the famous trade associations started writing their famous letters to me and to the producers of the show, protesting my lack of consideration in criticizing the presence in meat of a chemical that causes agonizing death via cancer. They eagerly pointed out that this poison reduced the cost of raising cows by a few cents a pound—although not necessarily the price of meat in the supermarket. I suppose that everyone who dares to criticize the poisons in our meat gets the same flurry of bullying letters. (By the way, trade associations of the world, please direct your threats to me personally at the address indicated in the front of this book. Include sufficient postage for a reply.)

Anyhow, the reason you eat so much meat and drink so much milk, eat so much cheese, gobble so much ice cream and gorge on other less-than-ideal proteins is that you are constantly nagged and threatened to do so. There is no American Soybean Promotion Council telling you to munch on soybeans if you want to be sexy. But the hog who lives on soybeans is far healthier than the blonde in the skimpy bathing suit who nags you to drink milk. Another few years on her milk and meat diet and she'll be posing with her hands folded in front of her to hide her fat little tummy. If she can still wriggle into her bathing suit, that is.

Your government nutritionists should know better too. Listen to what one expert said:

The Administrator of the Federal Security Agency, at a major food conference, remarked for all to hear: "Tortillas and beans are not any nation's traditional food. They are only the remnant poor folks can still afford."

Caramba! Every day 500 million people, rich and poor, sit down with gusto to at least one serving of tortillas and beans. Why? Well, they're smarter than the high-class nutritionists. Six tortillas and one-fourth cup of beans give them 14 grams of complete, top-quality protein with all the essential amino acids in a vitamin-and-mineral-rich, high-fiber package. That's the equivalent of almost 3 ounces of T-bone steak—and without the added chemicals. Oh yes, at about one fourth the cost. And that 14 grams of high-quality protein is nearly half the protein requirement of the average man. Not bad for a "remnant only poor folks can afford," eh, Administrator? And incidentally if meat, cheese, and milk prices keep going up, tortillas and beans may soon be the remnant only *rich* folks can afford.

Try another favorite dish of "poor folks": brown rice and black beans. One and a half cups of black beans and four cups of brown rice mixed together give you the same top-quality protein value as *19* ounces of steak. That's not too bad either.

Feel like a peanut butter sandwich? Be sure it's real peanut butter—not adulterated with sugar or mysterious "vegetable oil" and free from deadly aflatoxins. Spread about one-half cup of that on some homemade whole wheat bread containing three cups of whole wheat flour plus one-fourth cup of powdered skim milk. That will give you the protein power of a full pound of greasy steak.

But does that mean you should stop eating meat and drinking milk?

Hardly. But it does mean that you owe it to yourself and your family to take a good hard look at the prestige proteins you're paying such big money for. Milk is a good example.

It is true that milk is the perfect food—provided you're three days old and it comes from your mother's breast. Cow's milk is more a habit than a virtue. It's good for baby cows and, as I've pointed out, it's only so-so for humans. You may like its taste, but it has a lot of fat, not much in the way of minerals, and is so lacking in vitamins that it has to be "fortified" with cheapie synthetic vitamins. As a source of protein it borders on disastrous—a cup of milk gives you less protein power than a cup of lima beans or a cup of plain old brown rice.*

---

* Here are the precise figures: One cup of "fortified" milk supplies 28 percent of the limiting amino acid. One cup of lima beans gives you 34 percent of the limiting amino acid. All figures are based on the protein needs of a 160-pound man. The concept of the "limiting amino acid" is a way of grading proteins. The percentage content of the least abundant essential amino acid drags down the quality of the rest of the essential amino acids to its level, as we have seen. These figures are from *Amino Acid Content of Foods*, Food and Agriculture Organization of the UN, Rome, 1972, and Church, C. and H., *Food Values of Portions Commonly Used*. Philadelphia, J. B. Lippincott, 1970.

Maybe it's time to see a few $100,000 TV commercials where the big-league baseball player yells: "EVERY BODY needs LIMA BEANS!"

How about meat? Is that bad for you too?

Not necessarily. Meat is an excellent source of protein —along with fish and poultry. It only has a few things against it. First, it is much too expensive for what you get. Second, it tends to be loaded with dangerous chemicals like the carcinogen diethylstilbestrol, residues of DDT, pesticides, and all the antibiotics that are pumped into meat animals these days. You don't need those chemicals and you shouldn't eat them. Third, ham, bacon, and sausage products almost always (in the United States) contain sodium nitrate and sodium nitrite, which may form cancer-producing compounds in the body. Who needs to be done in by hot dogs?* Fourth, eating a lot of meat fills you up so much that you don't have any room for other vital foods such as fresh fruits and vegetables and whole grain cereals. Fifth, as we have seen, meat contains a lot of fat, and if you eat a lot of anything that contains a lot of fat, you get fat too.

In spite of all that there is a place in a normal diet for relatively small amounts of meat, fish, and poultry. Eating a pound of meat a day probably isn't that good for you. Eating a quarter of a pound of meat or fish or poultry probably won't do you much harm. Vegetarians aren't a bunch of wild-eyed fanatics. In general, they live longer and healthier lives than big meat eaters, but it takes a very special person with a very special point of view to be a vegetarian. If you like meat, fine. But just take it easy.

A good protein diet contains reasonable amounts of as many protein-containing foods as possible. Try a little bit

---

* We'll discuss the whole question of cancer-producing chemicals later on. However, it's worthwhile noting here that the major use of these chemicals in ham and sausage is to make them look nice and red—instead of the brown-gray they really are. Like putting lipstick on a corpse?

of beans, brown rice, whole wheat bread and whole wheat pasta, eggs, milk, cheese, fish, meat, poultry, and nuts. In the long run you'll be eating better, spending less, and living longer.

CHAPTER X
Sugar

How does sugar stack up as a food?

It's impossible to say because sugar—that is, *white refined sugar—is not a food*. It is a pure chemical extracted from plant sources, purer in fact than cocaine, which it resembles in many ways.* Its true name is *sucrose* and its chemical formula is $C_{12}H_{22}O_{11}$. It has 12 carbon atoms, 22 hydrogen atoms, 11 oxygen atoms and *absolutely nothing else to offer*. Refined sugar has *no* vitamins, *no* useful minerals,† *no* enzymes, *no* trace elements, *no* fiber,

---

* Does the comparison between sugar and cocaine seem strange to you? Let's look closely:

1. Sugar is a highly refined, white crystalline powder—so is cocaine.
2. The chemical formula for cocaine is $C_{17}H_{21}NO_4$. Sugar has the formula $C_{12}H_{22}O_{11}$. For all practical purposes, the difference is that sugar is missing the "N," or nitrogen atom.
3. Both are derived from common plant sources.
4. Both are powerful chemical substances producing strong physical and emotional effects.
5. Both sugar and cocaine produce psychological dependence but not true addiction.
6. Cocaine is not associated medically with any serious physical disease. Sugar is implicated in heart disease, obesity, diabetes, kidney disease, tooth decay, and blindness . . . to name a few.
7. Importing refined cocaine into the United States is a federal offense. Importing refined sugar into the United States is a federal offense.

† An infinitesimal amount of iron present as an impurity hardly qualifies as a "useful mineral."

no protein, *no* fat, *and no benefit whatsoever in the human diet.* Aside from that, it's fine.

But isn't sugar an excellent source of energy?

It certainly is—but not the kind of energy you want. Selling sugar is a big business, one of the biggest food businesses in the entire world. Sugar sales in the United States alone run about 32 billion pounds a year; at approximately 20 cents a pound wholesale, that adds up to about $6.4 billion dollars a year. Not bad. So the sugar industry has a whole slew of pressure groups (sorry, they are now called "public relations firms") to convince you that refined sugar is good for you. These front organizations have very classy names like "The Better Nutrition Seminar," "Food Utilization Council," and other slightly confusing aliases. They take big expensive ads telling you that sugar is your best source of "energy."

From the way the ads are worded, you might think that sugar gives you get-up-and-go, vitality, enthusiasm, you know, ENERGY! Nope, the only energy they're talking about is *calories!* It's not their fault if you misunderstood, is it? As a matter of fact, that tame tiger known as the Federal Trade Commission has slapped most of the sugar groups on the wrist for suggesting that refined sugar is good for you. The truth is that sugar will only make you fat—and even worse, if you're tired and lacking in pep, a good slug of refined sugar will only make you more lethargic and ravenously hungry.

How can sugar make you lethargic?

Easy. Sucrose, or refined white sugar, is a combination of two simple sugars, glucose and fructose. In the intesines there is an enzyme known as *sucrase* that quickly breaks down *sucrose* into glucose and fructose. The glucose is then absorbed into the bloodstream, with the excess stored in the liver. Glucose is the gasoline of the body and must be constantly available for anything that requires work, like operating muscles, physical movements, digestion, beating of the heart, and even thinking. As a result there are a series of complex mechanisms in the body to maintain the concentration of glucose in the bloodstream at a fixed level. That concentration averages about 100 milligrams of glucose per 100 milliliters of blood, which amounts to about one thirtieth of an ounce of sugar per quart. If the concentration of blood sugar goes much above that, a chemical called *insulin* is released from the pancreas to neutralize the glucose and bring it down to a normal level. If the concentration of glucose in the blood gets too low, glucose is released from the liver, where it is stored in the form of a substance called *glycogen*.

With that basic mechanism in mind, it's easy to see how a good slug of refined sugar affects your body. Let's say it's been a hard day at work and five o'clock is still two hours away. You remember the full-page ads about "sugar means energy." You believe it, so you drink a cup of coffee with a lot of sugar and maybe even wolf down a couple of candy bars at the same time. You've just shocked your body with about 3 ounces of naked sugar, and your blood glucose suddenly zooms up to 180 milligrams percent. You have given yourself "temporary diabetes," or more gently expressed—hyperglycemia. You feel weak, tired, and totally lacking in all energy. If you're lucky, your pancreas starts desperately pouring out insulin to counteract the overdose of sugar, and in an hour or so you start to feel a little better. You've probably spent about a dollar, drained your pancreas of precious insulin, and soaked up 750 calories that you don't need and don't want. In addition, the massive dose of insulin from your pancreas makes you unbelievably hungry. Feel cheated? You should.

But how did sugar get to be such a big business?

It wasn't always that way. In the beginning, sugar was about as popular in the average diet as hummingbird tongues—and much more expensive. Back in 1300 when sugar was first introduced to Europe from India, a pound of sugar would set you back the equivalent of $10,000. At a big banquet the king might sprinkle a few grains of the white stuff on his mutton chops. As time went by and production increased, the price began to drop. Giant sugar plantations were established in the West Indies, and sugar beets were planted in England. By 1850 sugar was cheap and widely available to poison the masses. By 1975 refined sugar became the most commonly used adulterating chemical in the processing of food.

Now hold on. What do you mean by "poisoning the masses" and "the most commonly used adulterating chemical"? Isn't that too strong?

If you like the truth, it isn't too strong. Sugar originally was used as a sweetening agent. For the past fifty years it has been used to *adulterate food*. Let's check *Taber's Cyclopedic Medical Dictionary*, p. A-26, for the definition of "adulterant": "That which adulterates or weakens a substance."

In most cake and pastry mixes you will find more sugar than flour. Ice cream and all the cheapie versions thereof, including ice milk, imitation ice milk, imitation ice cream, frozen dessert, imitation frozen dessert, have one thing in common: they almost always contain more refined sugar than any other ingredient, including "cream." How come? Because sugar is the heaviest common food ingredient available. And it's cheap. Cake mixes are sold by weight—it says so on the box so you won't think that the half-filled box is cheating you. (Isn't it?) A cup of flour weighs 100 grams. A cup of sugar weighs 200 grams. It takes about four and a half cups of flour to fill a one-pound cake mix box. You can achieve the same selling weight with two and a quarter cups of refined sugar. So food processors can get the same price for *half* the product. That's good for profits. Sugar is also used to adulterate breakfast cereal.

What makes you think that?

The medical dictionary says cereal is "edible grains." The label on a typical "cereal" box says "CEREAL." The label on the side panel of one of the most widely sold "cereals" admits that it contains 49.38 percent "sucrose and other sugars." By definition "sucrose and other sugars" must be an adulterant in breakfast "cereal." Any questions?

Sugar is also used to adulterate bread. Supermarket "enriched white bread" typically contains about 10 percent refined sugar. Its purpose is to make the product sweeter and heavier, since bread is sold by weight. It also covers up the awful taste of overrefined white flour and the various chemicals that bread is doped with. If bread is "enriched" with anything, it is "enriched" with refined sugar. Thus by any scientific standard, sugar is used to adulterate bread. You will also find sugar as a prominent ingredient in a lot of other foods where it really doesn't belong. When you make soup at home, do you add a slug of sugar? How about your mayonnaise? Crackers? Fresh vegetables? The food processors add sugar to all these foods. Sugar is also a prominent ingredient in each of the following "convenience" foods:

Peanut butter, baby food, pickles, spaghetti sauce, frozen dinners, frozen pizza, salad dressing, some instant coffee mixes, gelatin desserts, canned fruits, canned vegetables, tomato juice, hot dogs and other sausages, and those brightly colored powders you use to make imitation fruit drinks for the kids.

But isn't sugar necessary to sweeten those products?

You be the judge of that. Let's take a product most Americans use at least once a day. It's called by various names: "nondairy coffee creamer," "coffee whitener," and about a dozen brand names. If you don't want to put milk into your coffee, you dump this nice white powder into it. It looks a little like powdered milk and a lot of people

171

use it instead of sugar or cream. You know, they want to cut down on calories and all that. That's their first mistake.

Why is it a mistake?

Let's check a typical list of ingredients:

"Corn syrup solids, vegetable fat, sodium caseinate, potassium phosphate, monoglycerides, sodium silicoaluminate, sodium tripolyphosphate, beta carotene, and riboflavin."

That junk could come right out of Junior's chemistry set, but that's not what concerns us most right now. If you dump that stuff into your coffee to cut down on your sugar intake, you're in for a big surprise because it's basically sugar! "Corn syrup solids" is a sneaky way of trying to conceal from you the fact that the dominant ingredient in the product is a cheap form of refined *dextrose*, otherwise known as *glucose*. (Incidentally the "vegetable fat" is almost certainly junky coconut oil.*) One teaspoon of the "whitener" is about half a teaspoon of sugar and half a teaspoon of coconut fat. Yuk! The other chemicals are there to keep the concoction from turning brown, gumming up, or in any other way betraying its vulgar origin. Calories? About 12 per teaspoonful, or twice as many as you'd get if you used milk. The next time a waitress or airline hostess serves you that stuff in liquid or powder form—ask for real milk instead. You'll be doing yourself a favor.

A rapid review of some common food items will show how easy it is to work your way up to that 150 or so pounds of sugar† a year most Americans consume. (I don't

* If it's any consolation, and I don't think it is, food processors will soon be forced to tell you exactly what kind of "vegetable fat" they're putting in your dinner. It should be interesting to watch the results.

† Unless specified, this figure and all others applying to "sugar" refer to all the common commercial forms of refined sugar—sucrose, dextrose, maltose, lactose, etc.

eat any refined sugar, and you probably won't be eating quite as much after you finish this chapter.)

Cola drinks get about 100 percent of their calories from sugar. Sometimes mothers feel guilty about that, so they give their kids those powdered concentrates in the little paper envelopes to make fruit-flavored "ades." That's an improvement—they're only 98 percent sugar calories. Parents who believe in TV commercials promptly switch to a powdered breakfast orange drink—you know the kind I mean? That's nifty—it cuts the kids' sugar intake to about 95 percent of the calories involved. Okay—here goes. If you want to cut your children's sugar intake—as a percent of calories—it's better to give them a *chocolate bar for breakfast* instead of one of those nice drinks. He'll only be getting about 30 percent sugar.*

Tired of heavy sugary desserts like brownies made from a mix? Okay, switch to a popular brand of nice, light, fruit-flavored gelatin dessert. But don't expect to eat less sugar. Bite for bite, you'll get twice as much sugar in the fruit-flavored gelatin mixture. The brownie mix runs about 33 percent sugar—the gelatin dessert will ring the bell at *over 85 percent sugar*. Hope you have a strong pancreas!

But how did all this sugar-in-everything business get started?

Well, aside from being cheap and heavy, sugar is a good friend to food processors in many other ways. It masks the flavor of inferior and even spoiled ingredients. Lunch meat that you probably couldn't choke down otherwise seems almost tasty when it's heavily sugared. Fast-food chains love sugar. They dump it into cheap ground meat, hot dogs, fried chicken, pancakes, fish cakes, hush puppies, and almost anything else. If it's sufficiently doped up with sugar (and salt), most fast-food items taste almost good enough to eat. But the dirtiest trick of all, when it comes to sugar, is played on the most innocent and defenseless consumers of all.

* It's even better to just give him a real apple or an orange. But explain to him what it is, since it's not advertised on TV. Say: "This is real fruit. It won't hurt you."

Who is that?

Tiny babies. The gigantic companies who manufacture baby "food" know two important things about selling their product. First, they have to make the babies eat the "food." And that's a problem. Baby "food" is overcooked, over-processed, flat, and tasteless. That's why it's so mushy and pasty and awful-looking. But the secret ingredient is sugar. A good jolt of sugar makes sloppy baby vegetables and baby fruit and everything else even more acceptable to the baby—and particularly to the mother. If infants lap up the sugar-soaked salty paste that passes for baby "food," mother is happy too. She feeds baby fast and easily and has time left for her other endless chores.

But there's another commercial advantage to adding sugar to baby "food"—it makes for fat babies. Seventy-five years ago, tuberculosis was a serious health problem, and one of the obvious symptoms of tuberculosis was severe underweight. In those days fat babies were free from tuberculosis. Even though tuberculosis is now under control, modern mothers still like fat babies. And pediatricians weigh the baby on every office visit and note the weight gain on a little chart. Baby "food" babies are fat babies, and fat babies make for fat profits. But are fat babies healthy babies? No. Lean babies are healthy babies. Fat babies also make fat adults. Fat adults tend to be dead adults. Sugar doesn't belong in baby "food." There's only one place where sugar does more damage than in baby "food."

Where's that?

In infant formulas. There is a single nutritionally correct food for newborn babies: *human milk*. It is perfect in every way for mother and child. But there is absolutely no profit in selling mother's milk. There is immense profit in selling artificial imitation milks known as "infant formulas." They are cheap to make, keep indefinitely, and sell at very high prices. They make babies fat, they make life easier for mother, they make big profits for the companies that sell them. They are not good for babies.

But if they're not good for babies, how come they sell so much and how come pediatricians recommend them?

Because pediatricians are not experts in nutrition. They are good-intentioned, overworked men and women who daily fight a desperate battle against disease. Most of them just don't have the time or the background to dedicate themselves to good nutrition in healthy babies. Besides, the artificial-imitation milk peddlers have the upper hand. When a mother leaves the hospital these days in the United States, she gets a big box of artificial-imitation milk free to get her baby hooked—oops, started. One of the major international "baby-formula" manufacturers even hires women salespeople dressed like *nurses* to circulate among the backward African tribespeople telling them that mother's milk will make their babies sick and their only hope is to buy expensive artificial formula.

Let's just look at what's in the artificial-imitation milks and we can judge for ourselves. The basic ingredient in a typical artificial-imitation milk is nonfat dry milk from a cow. The number-two ingredient is usually lactose, a refined sugar composed of plain old glucose and galactose. The next ingredient in order of amount is usually our old friend coconut oil. Ugh! You try a tasty mixture of powdered skim milk, sugar, and coconut oil all mixed together for just one day and then you'll understand why your baby spits up. The rest of the long list of artificial vitamins and minerals are present in infinitesimal quantities. The only reason that babies drink formulas is they can't get out of the crib and go to the refrigerator to get something decent to drink. But infant "formula" and baby "foods" that are overdosed with sugar set kids up for worse things to come.

What things are those?

A lifetime as a sugar addict. Once the taste for over-sweetened foods has been imprinted during infancy and childhood, it remains forever. The average American child each year consumes over 20 pounds of candy, nearly 500 bottles of soft drinks, and 200 pieces of sugary chewing gum. Most adults don't eat anything unless it has been heavily sugared—all the way from wines, beer, and cocktails to snack crackers and frozen vegetables. (Yes, there is plenty of sugar in beer—it's called *maltose*.) That means bad news for everyone except the folks who sell sugar.

One of the most obvious forms that bad news takes is tooth decay. The cost of dental care in the United States currently is about $6 *billion* a year. And the rate of decay is so rapid that if all the dentists in the country worked twenty-four hours a day, seven days a week filling cavities, at the end of the year there would be just as many rotten teeth waiting to be repaired as there were at the start of the year. Looking at it another way, of each 100 men taken into the military service in the United States, on the average, military dentists do 600 fillings, 112 extractions, and 40 partial false teeth. The primary cause of tooth decay is refined sugar in the diet.

What makes you so sure of that?

Just start flipping through the medical journals and you'll be as sure as I am. One of the classical dental studies was done by the British government on the islands of Tristan da Cunha in the middle of the Atlantic Ocean between Africa and South America. Because of their isolation, for many years, islanders subsisted mainly on fish and potatoes. They did not consume refined sugar, and they were examined regularly by dental officers of the British Navy. In 1938, not one decayed adult first molar was found in residents under the age of 20 on the entire island. By 1962 the islanders were soaking up about a pound of sugar per person per week—about one third of what the average American consumes. At that time, half the islanders in the same category had rotting teeth.

But that's just one example, isn't it?

Yes. Want some more? There are over 100 almost identical studies in Ghana, South Africa, the United States, Britain, Australia, Sweden, Norway, and a couple of dozen other countries. In each and every case the results were identical: refined sugar rots teeth—fast.

Does it make sense to spend hundreds of millions of dollars for drinking water and toothpaste doped up with tiny amounts of a poisonous chemical—fluoride—when you soak your mouth in sugars that rot away your teeth? There's a safer and more effective solution: *just stop eating refined sugar.* And stop giving your kids food adulterated with sugar. Now what did they have for breakfast today? Was it one of those national brand sugar-coated cereals with all that nutritional gobbledygook on the label? The company that makes one so-called cereal says: "We're serious about nutrition." That luscious sugar-coated product contains three different sweeteners and by *their* calculations is 56.45 percent "sucrose and other sugars." Add to that *their* figures for "starch and related carbohydrates" —31.75 percent—and we get a cereal (?) that is 88.2 percent starch, sugar, and refined carbohydrate. *"Serious* about nutrition"?

There's another little problem with eating all that sugar.

What's that?

It can kill you. There is no doubt that *diabetes mellitus* —otherwise known as "sugar diabetes"—is caused by excessive consumption of refined sugar and, to a lesser extent, refined carbohydrates. Let's quickly review what diabetes is all about to see where sugar fits in as the basic cause.

When you consume refined sugar and it enters the bloodstream, the sugar level is regulated by a chemical produced by the pancreas called *insulin.* Insulin works almost immediately to reduce the blood sugar level and protect vital organs, including the brain, from sugar overdose. Excessive amounts of sugar in the blood can cause a condition known as *diabetic coma,* which can produce rapid and permanent brain damage and death. Excessive amounts of insulin can produce *insulin shock,* which also can produce brain damage and death. So the poor diabetic teeters through life on the razor's edge balanced between diabetic coma and insulin shock. But it's worse than that—and diabetics and relatives of diabetics have to face the reality no matter how unpleasant it may be, if they are to have any chance of overcoming their disease. Diabetes, for a great number of diabetics, means a life full of astronomical expenses, terribly unpleasant surprises, and a premature death.

No matter how carefully he controls his diet, no matter how conscientiously he takes his insulin, a diabetic may develop a massive infection from the smallest scratch, or he may see his fingers and toes and hands and feet become gangrenous without warning—and have them amputated. He is extremely vulnerable to high blood pressure, he has an immensely elevated rate of fatal heart attacks, and he has a good chance of becoming totally and permanently blind. Kidney failure is a serious hazard for diabetics. Many male diabetics can anticipate total and permanent sexual impotence—untreatable and incurable. Even tuberculosis is twice as common in diabetics as nondiabetics. Yet "modern" medical science has nothing to offer a diabetic except a prescription for a needle, a syringe, and a bottle of insulin. The doctor gives him a diet that no normal person can really adhere to and makes an appointment for another office visit in a month. That's the kind of treatment that has made the handful of drug companies which produce insulin fabulously wealthy at the same time it has made insulin addicts out of the estimated twelve million diabetics in the United States.

But at least insulin helps diabetics to live longer?

Maybe it does—in individual cases. But the statistics don't look so good. In 1900, according to British life insurance records, diabetes was in *twenty-seventh* place as a cause of death. Insulin was developed about 1922. By 1950 diabetes was ranked as the number *three* cause of death. Maybe that's because other diseases were declining and diabetes claimed relatively more lives? Not likely, because in 1900 the death rate from diabetes in the United States was 12.2 per 100,000. By 1971—almost three quarters of a century of "progress" later—the death rate from diabetes was 18.5 per 100,000 population. So in spite of the "modern" treatment for diabetes, in spite of insulin, in 70 years the death rate from the disease has *increased* 52 percent!

But even if you survive, diabetes is expensive. The average diabetic spends at least ten dollars a month for insulin, needles, and syringes. At least one doctor's visit a month with laboratory tests sets him back a minimum thirty dollars monthly. If he just has one insulin overdose or underdose a year with a hospital admission, that's another thousand dollars. So if American diabetics only spend half that amount—about $750 a year—that's still a tidy $9-billion-a-year industry.

So far, oral antidiabetes drugs have been disappointing, and a couple have been hastily withdrawn from the market. But there is a way to improve the health of diabetics that doesn't cost a penny and may actually help them to overcome the disease.

What way is that?

Well, first we have to understand that diabetes *is not simply a deficiency of insulin.* In fact diabetics tend to have more insulin available than one would anticipate. *Diabetes is the result of a pancreas exhausted by an extended overdose of refined sugar and carbohydrate.* There is so much proof for that statement that it is almost unbelievable it has been overlooked for so long. Summarized

179

below is the incontrovertible scientific evidence which establishes diabetes as the result of pancreatic exhaustion due to excessive sugar (and carbohydrate) consumption.

1. Diabetes is unknown in virtually every unindustrialized (wrongly called "primitive") society that consumes virtually no refined sugar and refined carbohydrates.
2. As soon as these societies begin consuming refined sugar and refined carbohydrates, they begin to develop diabetes. Usually there is about a twenty-year latent period from the start of heavy sugar consumption until the large-scale epidemics of diabetes.
3. As a corollary to number 2 above, the latent period in the average individual diabetic is also about twenty years—based on heavy sugar consumption in childhood.
4. The fact that diabetes has a *hereditary* component has been misused to insist that the amount of refined sugar one eats has nothing to do with the disease. That's not true. Listen to what the accepted reference books, such as *The Merck Manual of Diagnosis and Treatment*, say:

"Though a genetic component in diabetics has long been recognized, its mode of inheritance is still not clear. Epidemiologic data are most consistent with an autosomal recessive pattern, though a multifactorial inheritance mode has not been excluded."

Whew! That's reassuring! Actually I put my best translators to work on that little pronouncement and this is how it comes out in English:

"Doctors have noticed that the tendency toward diabetes tends to run in families but they don't understand exactly how. After checking a lot of diabetics, it might have something to do with recessive genes, but nobody *really* understands what's happening."

Okay, let's get back to reality. If your parents are big sugar eaters and you eat at the same table with them, you're going to get too much sugar too. Everybody has a different body—and a different pancreas—so some folks can handle more sugar than others. But if your Mom and Dad give you some yucky baby formula that is more than half sugar and bring you up on sickly-sweet baby food in jars, your chances of getting diabetes are better than ever.

If they follow that up with so-called breakfast "cereal" that is 56.45 percent sugar, what chance does a poor kid have?

Careful and responsible scientific studies have traced the development of diabetes in races who were once totally free of the disease as their consumption of refined sugar relentlessly increased. Those studies involved the following nations: Iceland, Israel, South Africa, India, Trinidad, Canadian Eskimos, Greenland Eskimos, Bangladesh, Cherokee Indians, Yemen, New Guinea, Polynesia, and several dozen others.

In each case the results were identical: virtually no diabetes until the group began to consume refined sugar in large quantities—about 75 to 100 pounds a year, or somewhat less than the average American soaks up.

5. The opposite experiment was done in World Wars I and II. Refined sugar and refined carbohydrates were extremely difficult to obtain. Both the incidence and death rate from diabetes declined impressively. If diabetes is a hereditary disease based on a lack of insulin, how can being deprived of just refined sugar and refined carbohydrates cure the diabetes in your great-grandparents that was supposedly transmitted to you?*

The white crystalline powder called sugar has caused the human race more suffering and more agonizing death than the white crystalline powder called cocaine. If you sell a pound of cocaine, you're a criminal and you go to jail for twenty-five years. If you sell a pound of sugar, you're a grocer and you go to Miami for two weeks in the wintertime.

---

* Back in 1949 a rather odd article appeared in a British medical journal suggesting that diabetes was caused by too much *fat* in the diet. The author reasoned that during the wars fat was also hard to obtain while carbohydrates were still prominent in the diet. He overlooked one vital thing: the only carbohydrates available were unrefined high-fiber carbohydrates which do not produce diabetes.

But didn't you say you were going to tell how to avoid diabetes and improve the health of diabetics?

Sure. But let me take a moment to give a vitally important disclaimer: *This book is not intended to give medical advice or suggest self-treatment. Diabetes mellitus is a serious disease which requires the constant supervision of a qualified physician experienced in the care of diabetics.* (Apart from the serious importance of the above, the publisher likes that because he thinks it keeps cuckoos from suing him. I think it encourages cuckoos to sue because their reflexes are triggered by legal language anywhere, even in a nutrition book.)

Okay, now let's get back to business. First, to save your children from diabetes, go into the pantry or the kitchen cabinets and throw out everything that contains refined sugar. Read the labels and if you find any of these words, trash the container and the contents: sucrose, fructose, glucose, maltose, lactose, galactose, cane syrup, corn syrup, corn sugar, invert sugar, dextrose, and anything else that suggests refined sugar to your mind.

Get rid of mayonnaise, ketchup, spaghetti sauce, all soft drinks, breakfast cereals containing sugar, all commercial pies, cakes, candies, cookies, snack crackers, gelatin desserts, and all the rest of the sources of hidden sugar.

Throw out all your imitation white bread unless the seller will certify that it doesn't contain any sugar of any kind. (Good luck!) In short, make your house as free of refined sugar as you possibly can. At the end of this chapter, we'll discuss the kind of sweetener that's safe to use.

Then go through exactly the same exercise with respect to refined carbohydrates. Get rid of everything that contains refined white flour. Dump all your white rice, white flour, and refined flour noodles—even the ones that are colored a nice yellow. Ditto for white spaghetti and macaroni and any of the other 50 varieties of low-fiber pasta you may have around the house. You can check the chapter on carbohydrates for more details.

But isn't that wasting food?

It you *don't* do it, the "food" will waste you. Speaking honestly and objectively, you are only throwing out distortions of food that have been adulterated with substances that aren't good for you. I know you're tempted to give it to poor people—but don't do it unless you have something against poor people. And above all, don't give it to the dog. For one thing, the overrefined junk you're getting rid of probably doesn't meet the U.S. Department of Agriculture standards for animal feed. It could get you in trouble. For another thing, dogs being what they are, yours just might eat it. You don't want to make your dog sick, do you?

After you have restored reason and sanity to your kitchen once again, put your family on a high-fiber diet.

Do you have any proof that kind of diet will prevent diabetes?

Well, it certainly won't *cause* diabetes. And based on overwhelming scientific evidence, it is the single most effective measure you can take to protect yourself and your family from that terrible disease. Of course, they are selling artificial pancreases now for about $10,000 plus installation and maintenance, but that isn't a solution either. If you already are a diabetic, have your doctor study the new and important techniques of treating diabetes with a high-carbohydrate, high-fiber diet. All it really involves is feeding diabetics a normal diet composed of unrefined carbohydrates and a lot of fiber. They don't eat any sugar on that diet—which is more than you can say for official diabetic diets.

You mean the usual diabetic diets give diabetics sugar to eat?

Sure—and plenty of it. The American Diabetic Association provides a series of diets* for diabetics which are used by almost every doctor in the country who treats diabetics. If you are a diabetic, your doctor might well put you on a 2200-calorie exchange diet which would allow you *ten servings a day* of the following items: ice cream, sponge cake, white bread (10 percent sugar, remember?), graham crackers, and corn bread. All these little goodies contain refined sugar and plenty of it.

That same list abounds in refined carbohydrates, including oyster crackers, saltine crackers, "round thin crackers," macaroni, noodles, spaghetti, breakfast "cereal," and mashed potatoes.

Some of the above items also have a good dose of sugar too. That so-called diabetic diet also allows up to eight servings a day of mayonnaise or French dressing—all of which contain more refined sugar than a diabetic should eat. But that's not all. The same diet includes eight servings a day of items such as salami, luncheon meat, ham, and hot dogs—all laced with refined sugar. You can top it off with peanut butter, which usually has a nice shot of the same white crystalline powder that can mean death for a diabetic.

But doesn't the insulin counteract that sugar?

No, it does not. Insulin merely prevents the sugar in a diabetic's diet from building up in his bloodstream and killing him then and there. Any diet that dumps massive amounts of refined sugar into the crippled body of a diabetic can't do him any good. A much better approach would be to eliminate all refined sugar from the diet—and all refined carbohydrate too. Then whatever insulin the damaged pancreas still produces just might be able to

* Krause, M. V., *Food, Nutrition, and Diet Therapy*. Philadelphia, W. B. Saunders Co., 1969, p. 302.

handle the sugar without the injection of expensive bottled insulin extracted from the pancreas of dead animals.

The dietary treatment of diabetes is based on the fact that a diabetic may produce as much as 60 percent of the insulin he requires. If he is given carbohydrates in the unrefined form, his limping pancreas can often do its job. But if he is overwhelmed with ice cream, sponge cake, and oyster crackers, he doesn't have a chance. It's like asking someone to move 500 pounds across the room. If he tries to do it all at once, he will pull muscles, raise his blood pressure, rupture himself, and maybe even get a heart attack. But if he moves it 25 pounds at a time, it's no strain. Many diabetics can still handle *unrefined* carbohydrates in reasonable amounts if consumed with generous quantities of fiber. In actual tests a high-fiber diet with unrefined carbohydrates has allowed some diabetics to discontinue insulin completely and has allowed others to sharply reduce the amount of insulin they require.*

Let's finish the discussion of diabetes with a short summary of the facts:

1. Diabetes is a common and increasing disease in industrialized countries, directly related to the consumption of refined sugar and refined carbohydrates.
2. Diabetes is virtually unknown in societies that do not consume refined sugar or refined carbohydrates.
3. People in these societies who start eating large amounts of sugar and refined carbohydrates start to get diabetes.
4. Insulin is not a cure for diabetes. Insulin is not even an effective treatment for diabetes. Insulin gives diabetics—and their doctors—the dangerous illusion that they can eat refined sugar and refined carbohydrates without hurting themselves.
5. Tests have shown that high-fiber diets free from refined sugar or refined carbohydrates can lower or eliminate the need for insulin in diabetics.
6. The best way to *prevent* diabetes is to follow the example of so-called primitive societies and eliminate as

* Kiehm, T. G., Anderson, J. W., and Kyleen, W., Beneficial effects of a high-carbohydrate, high-fiber diet on hyperglycemic diabetic men. *American Journal of Clinical Nutrition.*

completely as possible all refined sugar and refined carbohydrates from our diets—and especially from the diets of our children.

7. The most striking accomplishment of the "modern" treatment for diabetics is that the death rate from diabetes has increased 52 percent in the past seventy years! But it's really much worse than that. In 1900 there was no such thing as an antibiotic or a modern hospital. There was no urine testing for sugar, no million-dollar medical computers, and no superspecialists in diabetes. Usually a simple scratch or an ingrown toenail was enough to send a diabetic to the next world. Now we have everything, including insulin, and over 50 percent more diabetics die than at the turn of the century. Could it be the sponge cake and oyster crackers? The insulin?

8. Even the astronomical death rate for diabetics conceals the more terrifying real figures, since most diabetics die from strokes, kidney failure, and heart attacks brought on by their diabetes.

But doesn't refined sugar have at least some food value?

Here are the facts and figures, straight from the U.S. Department of Agriculture files. The comparison is be-

	Refined White Sugar (granulated)	Blackstrap Molasses
	(MILLIGRAMS PER OUNCE)	
MINERALS		
Calcium	zero	195
Phosphorus	zero	24
Iron	zero	4.6
Potassium	0.85*	836
Sodium	0.28*	27
Vitamins		
Thiamine	zero	0.03
Riboflavin	zero	0.05
Niacin	zero	0.57

* Don't be misled by the values for sodium and potassium. They are the most common chemicals on earth—found in everything. Even this piece of paper has more sodium and potassium than a pound of refined sugar.

tween an ounce of refined white granulated sugar and an ounce of so-called blackstrap molasses. Blackstrap molasses is used because unrefined sugar—misnamed "raw sugar" —is contraband in the United States. Actually unrefined sugar has more nutritional value than even blackstrap molasses.

So, there it is, folks. When you eat white sugar you are eating *nothing*.

But unrefined sugar doesn't seem to have very much in the way of nutrients, does it?

Whatever it has was put there by the Creator, and you can be sure there are other nutritional elements present which have yet to be discovered by our puny attempts at scientific research. And don't sneer at over half a milligram of pure natural niacin per ounce or 195 milligrams of organic calcium or that 24 milligrams of phosphorus or the 4.6 milligrams of iron. You get it all for nothing, it helps in the digestion of the sweetener, and it's more than you get in junky white sugar.

How come you can't get unrefined sugar in the United States?

Because unrefined sugar would sell at a lower cost than the refined cocainelike white sugar—and that's bad for business. In standard nutrition textbooks you will read the frightening statement that "raw" sugar is "filthy," full of dirt and bugs and other horribles. Of course, that's because of the way the sugar companies handle it and transport it. And they could clean it and sell it to you. Unrefined sugar is sold in about 200 countries in the world —and the people there are healthier than your children. But there's another quirk in the law in the United States— at the same time that *unrefined* sugar cannot be *sold, refined* sugar cannot be *imported*. That's because imported refined sugar is cheaper than American-refined sugar, and U.S. sugar refiners like big profits. At the end of 1977 they weren't doing badly; two of the biggest American refiners totted up a 250 percent and a 1120 percent gain in net income, respectively.* Not bad.

If refined sugar is so bad, why not enrich it?

Hmmm, I get it. As with "enriched" white flour or "enriched" white rice. Spend tens of millions of dollars a year to remove every possible bit of food value from sugar, then spend more millions putting a few cheap vitamins into it. Then label it "enriched" and get all your money back and more from the poor mommies and daddies who want to have their kids grow up strong and healthy.

As a matter of fact there was a feeble attempt to enrich sugar back in the 1960s. A small sugar company added iron, iodine, some of the B vitamins, and some vitamin A to sugar. That guardian of our nation's health, the Food and Drug Administration, acted swiftly. They seized the sugar, denounced it "misbranded," and took the shocked "enrichers" to court.†

"Enriched" sugar went off the market fast. But in the meantime there's always a new source of sugar just waiting to be discovered. If you smoke you get plenty of sugar in your tobacco—although you won't see it on the label. (Diabetics take note.) Most cigarette tobacco is about 5 percent sugar, cigars contain something like 20 percent sugar, and pipe tobacco can have *40 percent sugar* or sweeteners. Instead of smoking it, why not sprinkle it on your cereal? (Answer: Your cereal probably has too much sugar already.)

---

* Amstar and Great Western United.

† The accusation of "misbranding" is an FDA specialty. According to information I received, some copies of my book, *The Save-Your-Life Diet*, were sitting on the shelf in a health food store and less than 50 feet away was a display of bran. The FDA claimed that my book was "misbranding" the bran—or the bran was "misbranding" my book—I don't remember which. Apparently that 50 feet is the magic distance—like the 12 inches the chaperones used to insist on between dancing couples at the senior prom. I don't know whether they burned my books or burned the bran, but if they wanted a free copy, all they had to do was ask me. Oh yes, I suppose if this book is sold within 50 feet of *any* food product, the FDA will have another bonfire. Hmmm.

Well, if sugar is really so awful, how about artificial sweeteners?

Like cyclamates? Good luck. In a fit of sanity, the U.S. Congress passed a measure called "The Food Additives Amendment," which contains a single sentence that *should* be saving millions of lives. It is called the "Delaney Clause" and it states:

"That no additive shall be deemed to be safe if it is found to induce cancer when ingested by man or animals or if it is found, after tests that are appropriate for the evaluation of the safety of food additives, to induce cancer in man or animal."

The major food companies have launched a massive campaign against the Delaney Clause because they like to put things in your food that cause cancer.

But isn't that an irresponsible statement?

No. Diethylstilbestrol causes cancer in humans and test animals. Red #2 causes cancer in test animals. Cyclamates cause cancer in test animals. A few lesser-known but equally lethal food additives include

oil of calamus (a flavoring) : cancer of the intestines
safrole (a flavoring agent) : liver cancer
thiourea (a preservative) : liver cancer
diethyl pyrocarbonate (a preservative for drinks) : cancer

All these additives were present in your food in dangerous quantities—all cause cancer. Some of them were ultimately taken out of food—but only after a bitter fight by the food processors that used them and the manufacturers who sold them. There are almost 5000 exotic chemicals added to your food these days, and a lot of them are suspected of being capable of causing you to end your life in a cancer ward.

Now that cyclamate is gone—although the manufacturers and users are still trying to bring it back—the major artificial sweetener in the United States is saccharin.

Saccharin was discovered by Constantin Fahlberg and Ira Remsen in 1879. It comes from coal tar, a sticky, gooey, black tarry substance derived from coal. (Incidentally those cancer-causing food colorings also come from coal tar.) In 1907, under Teddy Roosevelt, the Board of Food and Drug Inspection was established. (That was the forerunner of the FDA.) Dr. Harvey Wiley was the first director and his first official act was to ban the use of saccharin in food as a dangerous chemical.

If it was banned, how come there's saccharin in my diet soda pop?

Thank tough-talking Teddy Roosevelt for that. He flew into a rage when saccharin was banned because, being a little pudgy, he liked to use it in his coffee. So he appointed a commission to reevaluate the safety of saccharin. And guess who was on the commission? A little man called Ira Remsen—who was the daddy of saccharin. Predictably the commission decided it was really okay to put saccharin in anything, and that's why it's everywhere. But it probably won't be there long. Maybe it isn't even there anymore. You see, up in Canada, where people apparently don't like the idea of dying from cancer, they reviewed the medical histories of people who used saccharin. After studying a group of 480 men, the investigators concluded that saccharin eaters were 170 percent more likely to develop cancer than nonsaccharin users were. That seems to be what the Delaney Clause is all about, isn't it? Anyhow I don't use saccharin, I don't give it to my family, and I tell everyone I like not to use it. You should make up your own mind.

But what kind of sweetener is safe to use?

That's not a difficult question to answer based on what we already know. The only types of sweetener that the human body is adapted to—based on its physiology, chemistry, and hundreds of thousands of years of adaptation—are natural, unrefined sweeteners. The ideal way to get your sweet taste is by munching sugarcane or sugar beets. Your jaw muscles will ache long before you can get fat or sick, and the cane or beet juice you get that way can't do you any harm. (Sugarcane cutters all over the world munch cane while working, and they don't have any of the sugar-caused diseases that refined-sugar users have.) If you don't live near a cane field, blackstrap molasses is the closest product available that is *almost* unrefined. You can't get "raw" sugar unless you are willing to smuggle it across the border. What is usually sold as raw sugar is refined white sugar dosed with molasses. Forget it. That goes for brown sugar and the rest of the imitations.

Honey is an excellent sweetener if it is pure and unrefined. A favorite trick of honey-cheaters is to dump refined white sugar into the honey, then cut the mixture with water. That isn't good for you. So uncooked, unadulterated honey is a fine source of sweetening. But that doesn't mean you can substitute 150 pounds of honey or molasses for the 150 pounds of sugar you eat every year. The idea is to eliminate as much sugar as possible from your diet and to use sweeteners as they were originally intended—in very small quantities as spices and flavorings.

But should I really give up refined sugar?

Only if you want to help yourself to avoid some or all of the following diseases: diabetes, obesity, heart attacks, dental decay, oral and vaginal infections, chronic urinary infections, and total blindness.

Let's look at it this way: If any food processor used a food additive that was one tenth as dangerous as we know refined sugar to be, that food additive would be banned by the FDA within twenty-four hours.

Think about it.

CHAPTER XI
The Ideal Diet

What is an ideal diet?

Let's get one thing straight right from the beginning: the ideal diet of the human race is the one that God has provided for them, period. That's it. Anyone who tells you anything else is trying to sell you his product—or somebody else's product. Since the first man set foot on earth, human beings have instinctively known how to select their diet correctly. *The great mass of food advertising is designed to compel you to distort your diet by eating expensive substitutes for natural wholesome food*. A black African in his tiny village eats a more wholesome diet than the millionaire in his penthouse on Park Avenue. A monk in Tibet eats better than a movie star in Hollywood. A farmer's wife in Spain eats better than a society woman in Miami Beach.

But what you said about advertising being designed to distort people's eating habits—isn't that overdoing it?

You be the judge. The biggest food processors in the United States are spending over two billion dollars each year to make you eat inferior chemical-laden artificial and imitation food—instead of what has been placed here by your Creator to sustain you. Let's check one of their

$80,000 full-page ads and see if we're overdoing it. The headline starts like this:

"Dear Blank Blank: Imitation this. Artificial that. Synthetic this. What's wrong with real food?"

Then in a masterpiece of condescension, they answer their own question: "Actually there's nothing wrong with 'real' food."

Thank you. Then the lies start:

"Or with any foods, natural or man-made, that you're likely to come across in the supermarket."

Come on, now. What about cyclamates, Red #2, saccharin, NDGA, BHT, coumarin, and dozens of other toxic chemicals that were (or are still) offered in the "man-made" food in your supermarket?

Farther on they ask the question: "Man-made foods: who needs them?" They promptly answer their own question:

"Okay. People need them. But why? Because, for one reason, they can save you money." Ugh! Eat junk to save money?

They continue: "Then, too, most man-made foods store for a long time without spoiling. . . ."

That is a reason *not* to eat man-made foods. The reason they don't spoil is they are so doped up with potentially hazardous artificial chemicals that they are virtually embalmed. One of the characteristics of wholesome food is that if it gets old it spoils so you won't hurt yourself by eating it.

But let's read their last alibi for man-made foods:

"Finally—and maybe most important—man-made food will help make sure the world has enough to eat."

Do they really think you are dumb enough to believe that feeding your kids imitation whipped cream out of an aerosol can will provide more food for someone in Vietnam? Will drinking a rotten sugar-laden soft drink give a child in Mexico a better diet? Will dosing you and your family with artificial chemical concoctions help anyone *anywhere* except the cynical men who make the phony food? You answer that.

But the most unbelievable part of the ad campaign is still to come. It's their comparison between a real orange and their artificial-synthetic-imitation-utterly-unbelievable instant orange drink. Here's why they say you should give your family such a product instead of a fresh orange:

"It's made with natural orange flavor. A 4-fluid-ounce serving gives you a full day's supply of vitamin C, and not even an orange can give you better vitamin C. It won't spoil quickly, and you can mix up as little or as much at a time as you want, without waste."

Would you like to know what that imitation instant drink *actually contains*? Get ready for a shock. (And remember that the ingredients are listed in order of quantity—the product contains most of the first listed ingredient.)

"Sugar, citric acid, carboxymethyl cellulose, sodium cellulose, natural orange flavor, sodium citrate, hydrogenated vegetable oil, tricalcium phosphate, artificial color, vitamin C, vitamin A, and butylated hydroxytoluene."

By weight, it is 13 percent cheap refined sugar, and 93 percent of the calories come from that sugar. It contains more carboxymethyl cellulose (made from waste cotton lint) than orange flavoring, and more cheap hydrogenated vegetable oil than vitamins. As a matter of fact, it contains *more artificial color than vitamins.*

An orange contains natural orange flavoring and vitamins—no cotton lint by-products, no butylated hydroxytoluene, and no awful hydrogenated vegetable oil. An orange also contains protein, fiber, calcium, phosphorus, iron, sodium, potassium, vitamin A, vitamin B₁, riboflavin, niacin, and 50 percent more vitamin C per serving than the "instant breakfast drink"—and all of it really natural.

What about the other claims for the "man-made" drink?

They are laughable—and by the way, "man-made" is supposed to sound better than "artificial" or "imitation," but most of the things that man has made haven't turned out that well. The atomic bomb, cyclamates, Watergate, and all the rest, for example. Anyway back to the claims:

"*It won't spoil quickly.*" What does "quickly" mean? Oranges don't spoil quickly either.

"*. . . and you can mix up as little or as much at a time as you want, without waste.*"

Well, you can eat as little or as much of an orange as you like without waste. *Who are they kidding?*

So if you want an orange, eat an orange. If you want a glass full of cheap chemicals and worthless refined sugar, just buy a jar of instant-artificial-imitation-synthetic breakfast drink. Good appetite!

What's the best time to start on an ideal diet?

The first day you arrive on earth. That's why women have breasts, and that's why milk comes out of them—to give babies the best possible start in life. Human milk is so good for human babies—and the cheapie substitutes are so bad—that almost every woman who really understands the difference will want to breast-feed her babies.

Let's look at a few of the most vital differences between cow's milk and human milk:

Human Milk	*Cow's Milk*
Formulated for humans	Formulated for cows
Clean, free, warm, fresh	Contains bacteria, expensive, cold, several days old at best
Maximum mother-baby contact	Maximum rubber teat-baby contact
Easy to digest—soft curd	Hard to digest—hard curd
Small amount of fatty acids	Large amounts of fatty acids (causing indigestion)

There is another interesting point: the digestive system of a cow is totally different from that of a human being. Cows have several stomachs, live on grass and hay, and are total vegetarians. If you give your baby the same diet as a baby cow, shouldn't you—in all fairness—eat the same diet as a grown-up cow? Tonight try a bale of hay for dinner and see how it sits on your stomach. Then ask yourself why your baby has colic.

But there are other far more urgent reasons to breast-feed human babies.

What are those?

Human milk is not the same from one day to another. The formula and composition change from moment to moment to provide the maximum growth and protection for your baby. Cow's milk is "dead milk," in the sense that it is stale and devoid of the enzymes and antibodies that human babies need.

For the first two or three days after a baby is born, the mother secretes a substance called *colostrum* by doctors and *first milk* by mothers. That colostrum can mean the difference between health and disease, between life and death, in a baby.

Colostrum is loaded with substances called *immunoglobulins* which actually provide immunity against disease. (Doctors classify them as *IgA, IgG, IgM,* etc.) In mother's milk in the very earliest days of life a baby gets instant protection from these dread diseases: poliomyelitis, dysentery due to the deadly *E. coli,* other Enterobacteriaceae infections, many viral infections, staph infections, and influenza.

After the baby receives his original dose of immunity, the amount of immunoglobulins slowly decreases, only to increase later on. But breast-feeding gives a baby much more protection than even that.

What other kind of protection does he get?

Well, he also gets all the antibodies and immunity that his mother has acquired throughout her life, since her antibodies are passed to him in her milk. Remember that the raw material of milk is blood, and the antibodies in the blood pass into the mother's milk. In a kind of gruesome joke, a baby brought up on cow's milk gets antibodies against calf scours, listeriosis, gallsickness, and bovine encephalomyelitis. He won't catch anything from a cow. But if a human epidemic comes, he will be defenseless.

In addition there is a secret weapon peculiar to mother's milk that even most doctors don't know about. It is called *diathelic immunity*. It works like this:

Suppose you are breast-feeding your baby and a visitor brings him an infection that you have never had. The bacteria pass through the baby's body, into his saliva, and into the mother's breast where it provokes the production of antibodies. In the next dose of milk, the baby gets precisely the antibodies he needs to fight his new infection. Thus the human breast constantly adapts to new threats, and it functions to constantly protect the baby. Don't expect anything like that from the waxy milk carton in your refrigerator. As a matter of fact, don't expect anything much from that heavily processed cow juice—but more about that in a few pages.

But if cow's milk is so bad, how about giving your baby a special formula?

You mean the phony-artificial-imitation milk they peddle in every drugstore and supermarket? Good luck! Since most of these products are basically cheap dried skim milk, they have all the disadvantages of cow's milk plus awful refined sugar and greasy vegetable fat. And check the prices—some of them cost more than champagne.

Cow's milk—from the dairy and in baby formulas—is one of the primary causes of allergies in babies. So many apparent respiratory infections in babies are nothing more than allergies to cow's milk. No baby was ever allergic to mother's milk—that's for sure.

To put things in their proper perspective, let's see what internationally respected nutrition experts say about feeding "formula":

"It is important to realize, however, that synthetic milk—no matter how nutritionally perfect or economical it may be—cannot take the place of colostrum for the first few days, and of sound management, sanitation, adequate equipment, and proper nutrition."*

And that paragraph, my friends, refers to feeding *horses*. If your horse gets sick, you can shoot it. And if your baby gets sick . . . ?

When everything is considered, artificial or imitation feeding of human babies has been a colossal flop for mothers and babies alike. (The milk and "formula" sellers have profited beyond their wildest dreams.) Farm animals such as calves and piglets cannot thrive on artificial feeding—they need their mother's milk. Human babies fed on breast milk have almost 100 percent freedom from intestinal infections, far fewer respiratory infections, and almost total immunity to allergies.

What if a mother can't nurse her baby?

Almost any mother can nurse her baby if she knows how to go about it. Any mother who wants to learn all the tricks should get in touch with the dedicated and determined ladies who make up a group called *La Leche League International.* They feel the way I do—only more so. Their address is 9616 Minneapolis Avenue, Franklin Park, Illinois 60131. Tell them I sent you.

What do you feed a baby after he's finished with the breast?

Ideally most babies should be breast-fed at least six months. Then it's time to give solid food—but *not* the kind that comes in jars and cans. Commercial baby foods are an insult to any baby. If you don't believe me, read the labels. Most of these products consist of small amounts of vegetables or fruits mixed with tapioca or "modified starch" to make the watery mess look thick. Many of them are doped up with refined sugar and are massively salted. The food is overcooked, the enzymes are totally destroyed, the prices are outrageous for a few spoonfuls of pap, and

* *Merck Veterinary Manual,* 2nd ed. Rahway, N.J., Merck & Co., 1961, p. 775.

it tastes awful. One of your baby's few pleasures in life is eating—don't cheat him out of it. (If you think that baby food tastes good, try it. Yuk!)

Just feed your baby what you eat yourself. For example, take some boiled potato and put it in your blender with a little liquid and then give it to baby. (Add a teeny-weeny bit of salt if it's necessary. But only a pinch of a pinch.) You can do the same with beans, carrots, squash, peaches, apples, bananas, and almost anything else. You can also liquefy chicken or meat, and anything else that baby should be eating. It won't cost you a cent more, because baby will be eating the same food as you. What you save on jarred and canned baby food will pay for your blender ten times over. And besides, your kitchen has more love than a baby food factory, doesn't it?

As your child grows up, you should guard him from the massive mountains of garbage disguised as food that school and supermarket are bound to inflict on him.

What do you mean by that?

I mean *you* should be in charge of your child's diet—not the candymaker, the breakfast "cereal" maker, the soda pop bottler, and the cupcake peddler. Twenty years from now—or next month—when your child gets diabetes, where will *they* be? When your cute little girl is swollen by obesity, will the junk-food sellers dry her tears? Will the sugar peddlers pay the dental bills? I don't think so. Soda pop, bagged snacks, candy, commercial ice cream, commercial pastries, commercial desserts, boxed breakfast "cereals," chewing gum, and all the rest will hurt your child—and you. They displace real food from the diet, damage the digestive system with their high content of refined sugar and refined flour, and steal vast amounts of money from your pocket. Aside from that, they're fine. But keeping your kids from being harmed by inferior over-processed food isn't easy.

Why do you say that?

Because junk-food pushers are worse than dope pushers. They even work the corridors of the nation's schools unchallenged. The U.S. government has a vast program of school lunches that costs taxpayers nearly three billion dollars a year off the top. But that's only the beginning, because the food comes from the federal farm price-support program where the government buys food from farmers at elevated prices to keep the costs high at the supermarket. (That's why they call it "price support.") The food is so rotten that an estimated one third is left on the kids' plates to be thrown away.* That's a mere billion dollars yearly in the garbage can. This food is things like canned beef chunks, canned sugared peaches and pears, "sodden canned hamburgers, mealy with textured vegetable protein," "limply breaded fried chicken," "pulpy fish," and "poultry below any government grade and in worse shape than products with deformities, bruises, and broken bones."†

At least 20 percent of the schools use frozen TV-type dinners that are described as "smelly, tasteless, and tepid." And the joker is that those frozen messes cost the same as fresh wholesome food; the only difference is that the kitchen equipment for fresh food costs a little more to buy at first. But school administrators say they would rather spend the money on "education" instead of better food. Do they want a generation of well-educated invalids?

But are the school lunches actually that bad?

You be the judge. Here's a sample menu taken from a "progressive" big city school district recently:

LUNCH: canned spaghetti, canned peas with butter sauce, sweetened canned orange juice, "enriched" white bread, canned pudding.

Every item on the menu is overloaded with sugar—in-

---

* *Family Health/Today's Health*, Sept. 1977, p. 40.
† *Ibid.*

cluding the slimy canned spaghetti. Refined white flour is in the "bread," the spaghetti, and the pudding. Do your best to train your children to eat wholesome food—and send them to school to eat pig swill like that? No, I take it back. Pig swill is far more nutritious than the average school lunch because you make money feeding pigs. There's no profit in feeding children—if you feed them well.

Would you be surprised to learn that a lot of kids pass up the awful school lunches to buy candy bars and soft drinks from vending machines? The vending machines are owned and operated by the schools, and the profits go to the athletic fund. The money really should go to buy Seeing Eye dogs for the children who are blinded by the diabetes that the chronic overdose of sugar can produce.

Some schools have just given up and invited the fast-food merchants to take over the lunchroom. (They might as well have prostitutes teach sex education.) That's probably because of the slanted food industry comparisons that say a fast-food, hamburger-based meal is better than the average offering in the school lunch program. The county jail probably offers better nutrition, too, but we don't send our kiddies there to dine—yet.

Let's analyze the typical fast-food school lunch:

Hamburger with ground soybean derivative: 250 calories
Sugar-laden hamburger bun: 125 calories
Processed cheese slice: 120 calories
Dressing on bun: 100 calories
French-fried potatoes: 150 calories
Milk shake: 390 calories

That's a mere 1135 sugar-choked, grease-soaked calories —and that's only lunch!

The greatest offenders in the field of nutrition education are the public schools of this country. While the teachers wearily teach from pathetic and antiquated charts reminding children to "eat two yellow vegetables a day," the lunchroom is feeding them senile canned slops from the farm surplus program. Next week have lunch in your local school dining room—if they'll let you in. Go into the kitchen, talk to the cooks and see where the food comes from, see how it's prepared and see who prepares it. Unless you're in one of the rare school districts that cares about the health of its children, you'll stagger into the parking lot weak with nausea and despair. There's only one place where you will be fed worse than in the temples of knowledge.

Where's that?

The hospital. It is almost an ironclad law that when the eater can't protest, the quality of the food goes down. Weakened, helpless, sickly hospital patients are given the worst diets in America. Don't believe it just because I say it. Listen to the Chairman of the Council on Foods and Nutrition of the American Medical Association, writing in *Nutrition Today.**

He says: "I suspect, as a matter of fact, that one of the largest pockets of unrecognized malnutrition in America, and Canada, too, exists not in rural slums or urban ghettos, *but in the private rooms and wards of big city hospitals.*" That's what you might call starving to death on $150 a day. Exaggeration? In the rest of the article, Dr. Butterworth gives a few examples, like the 80-year-old man with gangrene of his left foot. The operation was a success but the patient developed scurvy and severe malnutrition—and almost died. Instead of eating from his space-age vacuum-formed plastic hospital tray, he would have had a better chance eating out of the hospital garbage cans—at least the raw potato peelings would have given him the vitamin C the hospital dietitian carefully excluded from his diet.

But you said "starving to death," didn't you?

That's right. Let's go to the next case. That's a 52-year-old man who entered the hospital for heart surgery, weighing 120 pounds. His surgery came out fine, but he wasted away to 88 pounds on the hospital menu and literally

* Butterworth, C. E., The skeleton in the hospital closet. *Nutrition Today*, March/April 1974, pp. 4–9.

starved to death in a mere 83 days. What the German concentration camps took two years to do, a modern hospital can do in less than three months. I believe the word the hospitals use is "progress." The rest of the cases in the report are somewhat worse. If you have to go to the hospital, just make sure you have friends on the outside to sneak in enough food to keep you alive until you can get home. (Maybe they should make edible high-protein get-well cards?)

But don't they have doctors and dietitians to feed the patients?

Sure. Would you like to see some of the sample diets? Here's one for patients with gastrointestinal illnesses: "Eggs, dairy products, potatoes, lean meat, poultry, and cereal."

Not too bad? Right, but it's from the veterinary manual for dogs with digestive problems. Here's the hospital diet for human beings with gastrointestinal illnesses:*

BREAKFAST:

Orange juice with added sugar
Cream of rice cereal (refined) with added sugar
Enriched white "bread" (10% refined sugar)
Jam (50% refined sugar)
Tea with sugar

LUNCH:

Canned cream of potato soup with butter
Sliced processed cheese
Potato with butter
Enriched white "bread" (10% refined sugar)
Jam (50% refined sugar)
One 8-ounce glass of cream

---

* *Merck Manual of Diagnosis and Treatment*, 12th ed. Rahway, N.J., Merck & Co., 1972, p. 1659.

DINNER:

Bouillon (from a bouillon cube—over 90% salt plus MSG)
Egg
Potato with butter
Enriched white "bread" (10% refined sugar)
Jam (50% refined sugar)
Artificially colored and artificially flavored gelatin dessert
One 8-ounce glass of cream

There are also three snacks on that official hospital diet: in the morning another glass of cream with soda crackers! (Yuk!) In the afternoon apple juice with added sugar, and at bedtime a raw egg with cream and added sugar. The whole conglomeration makes up a diet so nauseating that the average sick patient just doesn't eat it. The nurse will tell the doctor that the patient has "lost his appetite." She won't tell him why.

One of the greatest swindles in the world today is a stay in a modern hospital. You are charged up to $150 a day for room and board. (Tests, drugs, rental of the operating room, oxygen, etc., are all *extras*.) For $25 a day you can rent a superb modern and quiet motel room, and for the remaining $125 daily you can hire a fine French chef to come to your quarters, shop daily at the markets and prepare the finest and freshest foods available in the most appetizing way. You'd save money and get better faster.

The hospital that feeds you refined sugar, white bread, canned soup bouillon cubes, and frozen vegetables should be closed by the Health Department as a menace to the public health. Of course, you could always send out to a restaurant for your meals, although I wouldn't advise it.

Why not?

Because a lot of restaurant food is barely food at all. It is a carefully engineered "product" designed for maximum profit—not for taste or nutrition. Is "engineered" too strong a word to apply to the food? Well, don't blame me. There's a magazine that you'll probably never see called *Food Engineering*, and it's full of all the details about how to make real food into strange combinations of chemicals, gels, colloids, flocs, and other weird things. It's not for family reading—just for the folks that sell to restaurants, supermarkets, hospitals, and the like.

Generally speaking, restaurant food is full of "taste appeal"—that translates into plenty of salt, refined sugar, and MSG. It has excellent "keeping qualities"—that means it's doped with preservatives. It is a "high-profit item"—that means cheap to the restaurant and expensive to you. There's even a new wrinkle called "portion control."

What's portion control?

More plastic. It's getting close to Christmas and you feel like treating the family. Take them to a high-class restaurant. You can tell it's high-class from the expensive carpeting and furnishings. Order Lobster a la Newburg for all four of you. Don't worry if it sets you back fifteen dollars each—after all, the place has a French name, the waiters are snooty, and you're out for a nice dinner. The lobster comes in good time—maybe a little *too* fast, but don't worry. It's salty, the sauce seems to cling to the few pieces of lobster meat like glue, and the lobster is a little rubbery. But don't complain because it's the wave of the future. You have just been portion-controlled—but good.

If you can force your way into the kitchen, you'll see a little shriveled man, standing in front of a little tiny stove. Behind him there is a big freezer. He reaches into the freezer, pulls out a little plastic bag labeled "L-A-N" ("Lobster a la Newburg"—what else?) and dumps it into a pan of boiling water. Six minutes later he takes out the bag, slits it open, and dumps the contents onto an expensive French china plate. The bag and its contents cost the owner $1.11. As the "defrosting technician" throws the bag into a pile of identical bags on the floor, we can glimpse a few more letters on the corner: "S: 1-4-C." That tells us that the "Lobster a la Newburg" was cooked on January 4 of this year in Seattle, Washington. Let's see, that's eleven and a half months ago. Hmm, does lobster improve with age?

But is it safe to eat in restaurants?

Sure. Only 42 percent of all contagious diseases in the United States are transmitted by food.* According to the U.S. Public Health Service, 32 percent of food-borne illnesses originate in the kitchens of restaurants and cafeterias. My calculator says that means about 14 percent of all people who get sick from food get sick from restaurant food. So watch your step. If you have to eat out, don't be ashamed to ask to see the kitchen. If they won't show it to you, then eat in a restaurant where they will. If they have something to hide, it can't be anything you want in your dinner. Stick to simple food items, and if you have any doubt, ask if the food you order was made there that day —or in Seattle, Washington, last year. Order fresh hot food—not hash, chicken salad, old stew, or any other convenient disguise for leftovers. And . . . good luck!

What about convenience foods?

In the food business, "convenience" is just another weasel word. It means convenient for the seller, not for the buyer. You know the expensive breading coatings they sell to shake onto chicken before you bake it in the oven? That's a little bit of flour, a tiny bit of seasoning, and a lot of salt. You can make a big dish of it for a nickel.

And let's check the salad dressing—a quart of heavily advertised brand-name salad dressing will set you back about two and a half dollars (four 8-ounce bottles). You can make your own for the cost of some oil plus a few pennies' worth of vinegar and spices. Do you think the big food companies have secret ingredients that no one else can buy?

---

* Harkins, R. W.: *J.A.M.A.*, 202:6.

Well, don't they?

Well, they have some ingredients they would *like* to keep secret. These days most commercial salad dressing—plus magarine, mayonnaise, and sandwich spreads—contain a weird little chemical called "EDTA." Those are the initials it hides behind on some labels, although in many products, thanks to the permissiveness of your FDA, it doesn't have to be identified at all. Its full name is "ethylene diamine tetraacetate"—that sounds bad already, and well it should. The purpose of EDTA is to cover up sloppiness in manufacturing. In grinding, mixing, and blending, food processors contaminate your food with a lot of metal ions including copper, aluminum, nickel, and others. They don't do anything to keep that junk out of your food, but they don't want it to spoil the looks of, say, your mayonnaise or salad dressing. So they dump in some EDTA, which traps the metal and keeps it from being so obvious.

EDTA also traps calcium, iron, and other nutrients in your food and keeps your body from using them. In animals, EDTA causes chromosome damage by disrupting the total cellular metabolism. (Human beings, by the way, are considered to be animals too, remember?) The FDA is studying EDTA for "possible harmful effects"—don't they consider disrupting the metabolism of the cells of an organism "harmful"? They should be through with their studies about the turn of the century.

One "secret ingredient" you can put in your food is "freshness." Another secret ingredient is freedom from the more than 5000 powerful chemicals that food processors routinely dump into your daily diet.

But isn't everything a chemical?

Yes, everything is a chemical—or a combination of chemicals. That includes your body, the paper in this book, your shoes, and what your doggie does on the rug. But you wouldn't want to eat any of those things in your daily diet, would you?*

The giant food processors have a wonderful line of double-talk that goes like this: "You don't like us to put chemicals in your food, folks? Well, tough luck, because everything is a chemical, including the food itself. So, if you don't like it, lump it!"

To anyone who is so bold as to suggest that some of the chemicals they dump by the ton into your children's snacks are poisons, they snarl: "You think cyclamate is a poison? Well, anything is poisonous if you eat too much of it—even table salt. So shut up and drink your cyclamate."

Isn't that a little bit exaggerated?

I don't think so, but let's check the processors' ads and you be the judge. Here's the start of a full-page ad that runs in the ladies' magazines:

"People Are What They Eat. So why should I eat propylene glycol monostearate?"

That's a good question. Then the ad goes on to state that propylene glycol monostearate is really just an "additive," not a nasty chemical. Do we really think that changing the name really changes reality? (Did calling the killer squads in Vietnam "pacification teams" make things any better?)

Then the folks who put all those chemicals—sorry, "additives"—in your food explain why they do it:

---

* That's not as farfetched as it might sound. Your United States Department of Agriculture has a wonderful idea. It suggests shoveling up chicken manure and forcing chickens to eat it. If you starve the poor critters long enough, they'll eat almost anything. They are also feeding chicken manure to dairy and beef cattle as 30 percent of their diet. There are a few little problems, of course. Since a cow's diet flavors the milk, the cows give milk that smells and tastes like chicken manure. Oh, well, they can do something about that, and as a matter of fact they have taken the first step. It's no longer called "chicken manure." It is officially the miracle ingredient "DPW"! (That stands for "dried poultry waste.") Don't be surprised if you see it soon on TV commercials: "Dee-Pee-Double-You! Costs less! Taste best! It's-the-Doo-Doo-Just-for-You!" (*Food Chemical News*, May 13, 1974.)

"Some foods would spoil without additives, some foods would discolor, some foods would lose their flavor without them . . ."

Does that sound like a lie? It should. It is. *Fresh* foods don't spoil, discolor, or lose flavor if you eat them fresh. Then the ad goes on to artificial flavoring—with more double-talk:

"If it weren't for flavoring additives [notice that the advertising agency sharpies never say artificial flavoring] you might have to do without your favorite flavors!"

That's a laugh. For 50,000 years the human race had plenty of flavors—without rotten artificial chemical additives. Then the forked-tongue comes out:

"Your favorite flavor might become obsolete. There is not enough vanilla in the world to meet the demand for vanilla-flavored foods."

Does that scare you? It shouldn't. The solution is easy: plant more vanilla beans. Food processors don't like to use real vanilla because it raises their costs by fractions of a penny per package. They use poisons instead—like "vanillin."

Vanillin is an artificial flavor made from the waste slop in the manufacture of wood pulp. If you feed a mouse one twentieth of an ounce of vanillin for each pound of his body weight, you will have a very dead mouse—and very quick. That's about 2.5 ounces of vanillin for a 50-pound child. Vanillin is found in chocolate bars, ice cream, soda pop, bakery goods, candy, and thousands of other things your kids eat every day.

But doesn't the FDA test all these chemicals?

Ah, you have been reading the ads. The suede-shoe boys from Madison Avenue go on to say:

"The U.S. Food and Drug Administration has established complex and thorough regulations for the safe use of additives."

That is nothing more than a sick joke. That's the same FDA that approved cyclamates, Red #2, cancer-causing DES in your meat, cancer-causing nitrates and nitrites in your diet, brominated vegetable oil in your soft drinks, and dozens of other proven dangerous chemicals in your daily diet.

Let's take a look at the "complex and thorough regulations for the safe use of additives." Back in 1968 the FDA set up a list of chemicals called the "Generally Recognized as Safe" list (known as GRAS for short). These chemicals were instantly declared harmless because they had been used in foods before and no one had died from them—instantly. They included items such as sugar, salt, starch, and about 800 more. Food processors were allowed to use *any* GRAS chemical in unlimited amount and without prior permission.

Here are a few of the present and former members of the GRAS list—with their Generally Recognized as *Unsafe* side effects:

MSG: *brain damage.* Saccharin: *cancer of the bladder.* BVO (fruit and citrus soft drinks): *degeneration of the heart and testicles.* Ammoniated glycyrrhizin (licorice flavoring): *high blood pressure.* Plus carob bean gum, gum tragacanth, benzoic acid, sodium benzoate, and BHA—all suspected by the FDA itself.

The "complex and thorough regulations for the safe use of additives" also allow the unlimited use of allyl heptalate, a totally unnecessary imitation pineapple flavor. In one little feeding test, that "additive" slew 100 percent of the dogs who were fed it. Then there's gamma valerolactone, another imitation vanilla flavor. In an official FDA study, rats eating the chemical had a mere 1300 percent more cancer than rats who didn't. You and your kids have probably swallowed some of both these goodies this week already.

But aren't those feeding tests crazy? I mean, you'd have to eat pounds and pounds of those chemicals before they'd do you any harm, and there's only a tiny bit in what you eat.

I know what you mean. Like the newspaper stories that snickered about the saccharin tests, saying you'd have to drink 800 cans of diet soda a day to get the same amount of saccharin that gave the rats cancer? That makes all the serious scientists in the country look like a bunch of nincompoops, doesn't it? But they're not—and here's why:

Suppose you gave your doggie a cookie from the supermarket and the pup uttered a shriek of pain, went into convulsions, and died—right there. Would you eat the cookie? I don't think so. What if your dog ate the same cookies for a couple of months and then died slowly and painfully from cancer? Would you give those cookies to your kids? I doubt it. What if the cookies gave cancer to big white rats instead of dogs? Would that make you feel safer? I hope not.

Okay, let's take the saccharin story as an example, but it applies to almost every other dangerous food additive in the same way. Serious scientists discovered that saccharin in relatively big doses gives rats bladder cancer, and they suggested that Americans stop feeding it to their kids and themselves. A lot of other countries just as smart as we are already prohibit saccharin. It is not a necessary part of anyone's diet, and it doesn't really help diabetics or fat people. But it does help the soda pop bottlers and food industry, who sell five million pounds of it a year. So the full-page ads and planted newspaper articles started coming out claiming that you'd have to drink 800 cans of diet soda a day for years to get cancer. Look at those dumb eggheads! They don't know that no one drinks that much pop—and besides they've never met a payroll, and a lot of them look like Commies. Ha! Ha!

Then along came the Cost of Living Council, who said that prohibiting saccharin would raise the cost of living! That's the only smart thing they ever said—when you die of cancer the cost of living goes right down to zero!

Okay, now hang on, because things are going to really get interesting. Those rats got a high dose of saccharin because there is a biological relationship between dose and time. For example, a big dose of sleeping medicine puts you to sleep faster—and you stay asleep longer—than a little dose of sleeping medicine. A big dose of a cancer-causing chemical gives you cancer faster than a small dose. Do you want your kids to keep gulping saccharin while the rats sip it in tiny doses and the years go by while we wait to see who gets cancer first? Rats are used as a biological magnifying glass—they have a life-span of about three years, and we can identify dangerous chemicals in our food much faster that way.

Oh yes, one other little detail that you won't see in those sneering stories about 800 cans of pop a day. If you give saccharin to pregnant rats, their offspring have a much higher incidence of cancer than the parents. It seems that the cancer-causing effects are sort of concentrated in the next generation. Think about that if you are a pregnant mother guzzling diet soda with saccharin.

But what does all that mean to us?

It means this: 10 percent of the rats got cancer fast—consuming the equivalent of 800 cans of diet soda a day. In human terms that means over 2 million cases of fatal bladder cancer a year in this country. That would merely double the number of people who die in the country yearly. But by computer analysis, if you lower the intake of diet soda with saccharin to 8 cans a day, you can expect a whopping 20,000 deaths from bladder cancer a year. Besides, there is saccharin in ice cream, desserts, puddings, pills and liquid medicines, baked goods, canned goods, candy, cough drops, and those little pills you drop in your coffee, so you don't even have to drink as much as 8 cans per day.

The saccharin peddlers talk a lot about "risk-reward ratio"—that means you buy saccharin and take the risk. They sell saccharin and get the reward. Cancer anyone?

But all that stuff comes from experiments in rats, doesn't it?

No. The National Cancer Institute of Canada recently proved that in 630 normal human beings the ordinary use of saccharin—not 800 cans of pop a day—increased the incidence of bladder cancer 170 percent. The Canadian government responded by immediately banning the use of saccharin in that country. But no one will lose money there, because they can sell all the condemned saccharin-containing products to Americans and their kids. You don't like that? Well, why don't you do something about it?

But that's only one isolated case, isn't it?

Unfortunately, no. A chemical that kills or damages animals doesn't belong in your diet—in any dose—even if it's a "natural" chemical. Going back for a moment to the food processors' ads, we find one, referring to artificial preservatives, that says:

"What we do in many cases is use the same or similar devices nature uses to protect its foods. We use sodium benzoate . . . to retard the growth of molds and yeast. It's a compound formed from sodium and benzoic acid, both of which are found naturally in foods."

Sounds wonderful. Therefore sodium benzoate should be safe since it is formed from two chemicals that are naturally found in foods? Okay, I've got an idea. How about combining a carbon-nitrogen radical—a chemical naturally found in foods such as almonds—with the same chemical in the ad, sodium? That should be just as safe as sodium benzoate, shouldn't it? Let's feed it to the smart-aleck advertising man who loves us to eat chemicals in our food. Will he mind? His survivors might. That little combination has another name—it's called sodium cyanide and will send him to heaven, or wherever big fibbers go, in about nine seconds. And by the way, sodium benzoate isn't all that safe either. It causes serious damage to fetuses and is now under leisurely study by the FDA as a dangerous food additive. The FDA takes a big-brother approach to food processors and has dutifully approved a lot of chemicals that slowly poisoned those who ate them.

"Poisoned those who ate them"? Isn't that going too far?

Well, let's look at a *partial* list:
Your FDA approved such tasty winners as cyclamates, Red #2, a whole bunch of other deadly colors including

214

certain oranges, reds, greens, blacks, and yellows, cobalt in beer, dulcin, ethylene glycol (that's the antifreeze you use in your car radiator, by the way), NDGA, and Myrj 45. After letting you eat those goodies for years, they suddenly discovered that those chemicals were bad to swallow. A little late for some cancer victims, don't you think?

The FDA is now suspicious of a few more chemicals that you probably ate already today. They include: MSG, BVO, hydrogen peroxide, carob bean gum, benzoic acid, BHA, and dozens of others. They don't seem to be in any hurry, since the study project is budgeted for seven years, and they will tell you it's all right to keep eating them until the day they finally decide to tell you—*retroactively*—that they have been doing you harm. Then they have another cute trick. It's called "allowing the manufacturer to use up present stocks." That means the manufacturers and food processors are allowed to empty their warehouses into your children's stomachs even though the sluggish FDA has decided that a given chemical causes cancer, brain damage, liver damage, or blindness or whatever. That's so the big companies don't lose any money. What's a few lives?

What is this FDA anyway?

We'll cover that in the last chapter. Stick around.

CHAPTER XII
A Few Final Words

What is this FDA anyway?

Well, it's not a bunch of geniuses, I can tell you that. The leading lights are usually a group of past or future employees of the giant food processors who stop off at the FDA to make friends or learn the ropes. The director of the FDA is usually a political appointee with no technical knowledge of food or drugs. Some of the recent job changes in the FDA were really interesting. They went like this:

The FDA's General Counsel (chief lawyer who decides whom to prosecute) came from a big law firm who defends large corporations against FDA charges. The former General Counsel took a job with a trade association which represents giant food processors against the FDA.

The Director of the Bureau of Foods came to the FDA from a big cereal manufacturer who doesn't want trouble with the government.

The Director of the Nutrition Division of the FDA left to work for a major candy manufacturer who doesn't want trouble with the government.

The Director of Product Technology of the FDA came right from a major canner and frozen-food manufacturer who doesn't want trouble with the government.

Is it right for the man who yesterday was vice-president of a big cereal company to join the FDA tomorrow and

The Director of the Nutrition Division of the FDA left to work for a major candy manufacturer who doesn't want trouble with the government.

The Director of Product Technology of the FDA came right from a major canner and frozen-food manufacturer who doesn't want trouble with the government.

Is it right for the man who yesterday was vice-president of a big cereal company to join the FDA tomorrow and write the regulations that determine how much profit his company is going to make? (Even if he doesn't have stock in the company anymore, his wife might or his uncle might or his lawyer might.)

Can a lawyer whose former law firm represents the biggest food processor in the country really apply the letter of the law to the clients of his former firm, especially when he's likely to be going back to work for that same law firm—with those same big clients—in a year or two?

Now do you know why your food is dripping with powerful artificial-synthetic chemical?

Back in 1907 when the FDA started—under the name of the Bureau of Chemistry—there was a group of healthy young male volunteers who were fed all the food chemicals before they were approved for general use. They were called the "Poison Squad," and if they got sick and/or died, the chemical was rejected. Now the Poison Squad has been abolished. Well, not actually abolished. It's simply been expanded to include you and your wife and your children and 220 million other Americans. Thank you for your cooperation.

But are chemicals really so harmful? Aren't those just scare tactics?

I don't know about scare tactics, but when I read the food manufacturers' ads *I* get scared. Let's try this one on for size:

The full-page ad features a picture of a nice meal with the food items labeled to indicate which ones are laced with powerful synthetic chemicals. The text says:

"In short, all the additives we use have some positive effect on food—or else we wouldn't use them."

Thank you. Thank you for those noble sentiments. However, "positive effect" is a relative term. When we fire-bombed a village in Vietnam, it had a "positive effect" on the "military situation." It had a negative effect on all those women and children who were burned alive. What may be a "positive effect" to the food processor is the saving of a tenth of a penny on a can of awful imitation pudding. That's more money in his pocket. The negative effect is the cancer the poisonous chemical eventually gives all the little kids who eat the slop—mostly because it's advertised on kiddy cartoons on television. And you notice that those nice advertising men say a "positive effect on food"—not a "positive effect on the people" who *eat* the food. There's a difference.

Anyway, let's look at that picture which illustrates the "positive effect" of food "additives." The photo shows a piece of fried chicken with MSG. MSG causes brain damage in rats, rabbits, chicks, and monkeys. A lot of eminent doctors think it causes permanent brain damage in children too. Where's the *positive effect?*

An indistinct glob on the plate is labeled "butylated hydroxyanisole (BHA)." BHA is prominently on the "suspect list" for dangerous chemicals according to the FDA Bureau of Foods. Its sister compound, BHT, causes rats to be born without eyes. *Positive effect?*

Something that looks like white rice on the plate is labeled "thiamine mononitrate." Well, they can't fool us with fancy names anymore. We know that thiamine mononitrate is nothing more than dirt-cheap synthetic vitamin B_1 put in there because many years ago the government forced the rice processors to put back a tiny fraction of the vitamins they were processing *out* of rice by making it "white" instead of natural brown. Don't take credit for *that,* Mr. Big Food Company. But since you brought up the subject of rice, why don't you tell the nice folks out there about another "additive" you dumped into their rice? It's called talcum powder. The "positive effect" of talcum powder is to make the rice look even whiter and smoother. That's why ladies put it on their cheeks. But that talc also may contain asbestos, which gets into your body when you eat the rice and gives you cancer after a number of years.

Most housewives don't like to serve rice with talcum powder in it—with good reason—so they wash the rice thoroughly. Remember about thiamine? It's one of those water-soluble vitamins. So when they wash the asbestos-talc out of the rice, they also wash out the vitamins. *Positive effect?*

But the real danger of chemicals is this: The powerful synthetic organic chemicals that are dumped into your food by food processors *are not part of the normal human diet.* You consume on the average about six pounds of artificial chemicals a year, and many of them come from nonfood sources, to put it mildly. Most food coloring—the "U.S. Certified" kind included—comes from a gummy tar derived from *coal.* Other chemicals are derived from crude oil and benzene. Many food chemicals are simply very high concentrations of naturally occurring substances. But they can kill or injure in high doses or with years and years of use.

They are chemicals that you would never add to your food on your own, so why should you let some big food company slip them into your daily diet just to make bigger profits for them—at the expense of your health? That's really what it's all about. And the saddest part is that food processors know better than you do how much harm they are doing.

What proof do you have of that?

Their own ads—the ones you will never see. Here's an ad from a nifty little magazine called *Food Product Development*—you won't find *that* on your neighborhood newsstand. It's just for food-industry insiders. Here's a sample:

"Show your true colors the safe way. . . . Get out of the controversy over coloring. . . . Want coloring without carry-through flavor? Here it is. There's even an ingredient you *won't* find in synthetics. The satisfaction of being certain your colorants are safe."

You will notice that the big boys don't talk about "additives" and "positive effects." They talk about "synthetics" and "colorants" and—imagine that: "SAFETY"!

Other ads say things like: "It's time to come back to natural flavor!" and "There's no substitute for natural flavor!" That's what they tell *each other*. But they tell *you* how great it is to munch synthetic chemicals. They have to be lying to somebody, don't they?

But how can you be sure that chemicals in our food are really so dangerous?

You be the judge. Would you ask your children to sit down to the dinner table tonight and choke down six pounds of oily liquids and grayish powders composed of 5000 separate compounds including many known or suspected to cause cancer in animals and humans? Would you deliberately feed your kids (or yourself) six pounds of 8-dodecalactone, carvacryl ethyl ether, hydratropaldehyde dimethyl acetal, 2-hexyl-4-acetoxytetrahydrofuran, nonanoyl-4-dihydroxy-3-methoxybenzylamide, and 4995 similar delicacies? Well, last year you did—and this year you and they will consume more of the same.

What's wrong with that?

Two things are wrong with that. First, you're doing it to make life easier—and bank accounts fatter—for big food processors. Second—and read this carefully—*you are running a terrifying risk of giving yourself and your loved ones fatal cancer.*

Do you have any proof of that?

It's all around us—although you won't find it on the label of your favorite imitation whipped cream, cake mix, coffee whitener, or artificial-imitation-orange-flavored-synthetic-vitamin-C breakfast drink. You will find it in the muted warnings of legitimate scientific societies and alarmed researchers (the ones who don't work for the big food companies, that is).

Virtually every qualified scientist agrees that human diseases can be caused by synthetic chemicals in the environment.

The people of the United States are the biggest eaters of cancer-causing synthetic chemicals in the world. In the first five months of 1975, according to the U.S. National Cancer Institute, *the number of cancer deaths increased 5.2 percent over the previous year!* That monumental increase occurred in spite of all the advances of modern medicine, cobalt bombs, Space Age surgery, and all the rest. In 1900 the death rate from cancer in the United States was about 68 people per 100,000. By 1974 it had soared to 170 per 100,000. That's a mere 250 percent increase in the age of medical miracles.

But does that mean that chemicals in food cause cancer?

The proof is right there before your eyes. Our society has a large number of test animals who have been living with us for over a hundred years. They are almost identical to man biologically, anatomically, and physiologically. They include the apes, gorillas, monkeys, and similar species in zoos everywhere. In zoos they are exposed to all forms of environmental pollution except one—massive doses of synthetic chemicals in their food. These animals almost never die from cancer—because they aren't fed cancer-causing chemicals in their diet.

Why not?

Ask any zoo director why he doesn't give synthetic chemicals to his gorillas: "Why, don't you realize a gorilla can cost over two thousand dollars?" And your children? How much does a new one cost?

Cows and pigs and goats and sheep almost never get cancer—because they are almost never fed cancer-causing chemicals. Farm animals are too valuable. In 1975, *671,000 Americans got cancer.* That same year, *368,800 Americans died of cancer.* What were almost 400,000 Americans

223

worth? More than pigs? And cancer isn't the only hazard from food chemicals.

What else is there?

How about the almost ignored report of a routine industrial study by the U.S. government's National Institute for Occupational Health and Safety? You better sit down before you read this one:

In the past 25 years the average sperm count in American men has dropped to an all-time low.

Let's just think a moment. The future of the human race depends on the production of those tiny little sperm by the testicles—and, of course, the egg produced by the female. A man who has 100 million sperm per cubic centimeter of semen is considered fertile. Between 60 and 100 million is adequate. Between 40 and 60 million is okay. Between 20 and 40 million sperm per cc is an area of questionable fertility. Less than 20 million sperm "is usually incompatible with fertility." That means *no babies.*

Okay. Taking the minimum 40 million sperm count as "normal," the National Institute discovered that *"the percentage of men with relatively low sperm counts had almost doubled."*

More than a dozen synthetic chemicals commonly used in your food can lower the sperm count by depressing production of sperms by the testicles. But don't worry. Chemists for the major chemical companies have already solved the problem for you. Keep eating chemicals because their answer is simply to *lower the normal value for sperm production.* Then all those sterile men will *officially* have normal sperm counts. But they won't be able to make babies. Has the world gone crazy?*

---

* Mean Sperm Counts in American Men Have Dropped. *Wall Street Journal*, Oct. 13, 1977, p. 36.

Okay, I'm convinced. But what do we do about it?

We stop eating food that contains dangerous synthetic chemicals. Basically that amounts to not eating anything that has an ingredient that even sounds like it came from a laboratory instead of a kitchen. If you don't understand what it is, don't buy it. And don't be fooled by some sucker labels that say "BHA and BHT added to preserve freshness." That's a new tactic of food processors to sell you alibis with their chemicals. If they can't get it to you fresh without artificial-synthetic chemicals, you don't want it. And you don't want "chemicals with an explanation"—you just don't want chemicals in your food at all. Okay?

Now let's get down to cases. Don't use soda pop in any form. By law the FDA allows it to contain, among other things:

1. *Ethyl alcohol*, the same alcohol that makes up whiskey. There's less alcohol in a cola drink than in a glass of booze, but you don't want your 5-year-old to drink *any* alcohol, do you?
2. Acids—acetic acid (otherwise known as vinegar), adipic acid, citric acid, gluconic acid, and malic acid, among others.
3. BHA, BHT, sodium alginate, propyl gallate, and methyl paraben—all unexciting in the tiny tummies of kiddy pop-drinkers.
4. Caffeine—you don't let your children guzzle strong coffee, do you? No, because caffeine isn't good for little kids. But a cola drink is fine? No. Eight ounces of coffee contains about 90 milligrams of caffeine. Eight ounces of cola contains up to 72 milligrams of caffeine. Now do you understand why Junior runs around the house all day like a rocket and why it takes two hours to put him to bed? The FDA can take another bow there too. They require all cola drinks (and "pepper" drinks too) to contain caffeine but not to show that potent ingredient on the label. Nice going.

Here are a few more reasons not to buy soft drinks:

1. Soda pop is outrageously expensive. You pay about 65 cents a quart currently for a product that is 99 percent water.

2. It is loaded with sugar—the average 12-ounce cola drink has 150 calories. all due to sugar. It is 10 percent sugar by weight, and that means about 7 teaspoons (over an ounce) of sugar per bottle. The sugar is cheap, rotten refined sugar that can only do you damage— diabetes, obesity, tooth decay, and all the rest. Diet pop has all the disadvantages of regular pop except the sugar—plus one more hazard. The substitute for sugar can do you in mighty fast too. But wait—if saccharin is banned, they will probably put sugar back into diet pop —corn sugar this time. Cheap and sickly sweet.

3. Citrus-flavored drinks—orange, lemon, lime—which are second in popularity only to cola drinks, contain that time bomb called BVO. BVO is the brominated vegetable oil we have mentioned before. It is composed of olive, sesame, corn, or cottonseed oil doped up with a nasty little poisonous chemical called bromine. Its only function in soda pop is cosmetic. It makes the pop cloudy so it doesn't look like what it is: water from the tap with a little flavoring and a lot of sugar. BVO has a little problem: if rats are fed one half of one percent of their diet as BVO for a mere 80 days, they suffer damage to their heart, liver, thyroid gland, kidneys, and testicles. Would you like to take the chance that your heart and testicles are stronger than a rat's? That's what you're doing if you drink most of the noncola soft drinks. But don't worry. BVO is illegal for such use in Belgium, Sweden, Britain, and many other countries. It is also prohibited in the United States. since it was finally removed from the "Generally Recognized as Safe" list. But it's *still* in your pop because the FDA is allowing the manufacturers to keep using it for a few more years anyhow. Oh, well.

What else should we keep away from?

Don't buy most "snack foods" such as cheese zippies, onion-flavored knock-knocks, mini-pizza yummies, and all the rest. They are usually combinations of three popular poisons: refined white flour, refined white sugar, and cheapie vegetable oil. They usually contain a whopping dose of chemicals as well as BHA/BHT in abundance. They are also outrageously expensive. You can make much better for less. Another alternative is to buy good natural snacks such as nuts, pumpkin seeds, sunflower seeds, and the rest of the real snacks. Get them raw if possible, otherwise dry-roasted. Don't buy them soaked in grease or fried in oil or colored red like some pistachio nuts. Roasted soybeans or garbanzo beans are also excellent.

But sit down and do some calculations first. You can't afford to buy junk snacks. The finest pistachio nuts or cashews will cost you less than chemical-laden synthetic snacks. The "imitation foods" are expensive and they don't fill you. The real foods may command high prices but they fill you and nourish you.

That's a good point. Can I really afford the "ideal diet"?

I think the real issue is: "Can you afford anything else?" You don't transport your family in a jalopy with no brakes and slippery-smooth tires, do you? You don't take your children to a cheap doctor in a dirty back-street office, do you? You don't live in a rat-infested slum with cockroaches running over the dinner table, do you?

Of course not. But when it comes to food, do you really try to save money by buying anything but the best? Your body is made up of just what you put into it—no more and no less. Every penny you spend on absolutely fresh top-quality food is an investment in health and strength and happiness. Every mouthful of junk food works to destroy your mind, your body, your health, and your appearance.

Have you ever stopped to think why many television

227

and film stars are so-called health-food nuts? It's easy. Their face (and body) is their fortune. Fresh wholesome food is the only way for them to preserve what they have. (We'll say a word about "health foods" a few pages farther on.)

What about other soft drinks?

They call them "soft drinks" because most of them will make *you* soft—in the stomach and in the head. Fruit "ades," drinks, punches, and the like are mostly water and refined sugar at high prices. Usually it works out like this:

"Fruit juice drink" can only be 50 percent water. (Big Deal!)

"Fruit ade" can be 75 percent water.

"Fruit punch" can be 90 percent water.

"Fruit-flavored drink" can be almost anything it pleases —more than 90 percent water.

It isn't worth it. If you want some juice, squeeze it yourself. But remember, you're much better off eating the whole fruit and drinking some water. Fruit juice lacks the vital fiber that keeps you healthy.

What about alcoholic beverages?

Most people think that the alcohol in alcoholic drinks is what does you the most harm. Well, alcohol does do you harm—just check your local skid row or charity hospital or police station to see how neatly alcohol destroys the human mind and body. And remember, all those derelicts were once happy little kids, laughing and running around. (And some of them *were* successful lawyers, doctors, congressmen, and public officials.) But the misery of alcoholism is another story. This story is about the other poisons they pop into your drinks, poisons that make a Mickey Finn seem like a health food.

How come?

Well, hang on to your hat. Labeling of alcoholic beverages is *not* controlled by the FDA. The Internal Revenue Service is in charge of that, and they don't require the booze makers to put the ingredients on the label. Most of the chemicals in your booze are carefully guarded trade secrets—for reasons that will become obvious in the next few lines.

Your bottle of beer can contain such surprising things as artificial coloring, propylene glycol alginate, our old friend EDTA, and heptyl paraben. Beer used to contain the metal cobalt just to keep the foam down. It also kept beer drinkers down, killing very quickly more than fifty beer lovers before it was banned.

But don't worry, additives in beer are under study by the FDA. Just hang in there until they get around to telling you what you shouldn't have been drinking all this time.

Wine is becoming more popular these days, and there is an official list that restricts winemakers to a mere seventy synthetic chemicals in their product. Wine can contain sulfur dioxide, copper sulfate (that's what you pour down the sewer to kill tree roots), and a little gem called "polyvinylpolypyrrolidone." That's closely related to PVC or polyvinylchloride, the chemical that has caused so many deaths in humans from liver cancer. Here's to you!

Oh yes, one other little detail. Until 1971 beer and winemakers were adding a little nothing called diethyl pyrocarbonate (DEPC) to their product. It was supposed to kill germs and then bubble away. (I thought the food processors were supposed to keep their places clean so there *wouldn't be* any germs in the stuff they sell to eat and drink.) DEPC did that, but it also produced a by-product—right there in the bottle—called "urethan." Everyone agrees that urethan is a powerful cancer-producing agent. It doesn't belong in your beer, in your wine, or in your body. Since it's not on the label, do you know if it's still in your drink?

What about milk?

I'm glad you asked. One of the greatest frauds ever inflicted on the American public is homogenized milk. Does that sound like heresy? Once again, let's consider the facts. When homogenization was introduced in the 1930s it was "sold" as a way to nourish your children better. "Why skim the cream off the top of your milk bottle to put in your coffee when we'll mix it all up for you and your kids can get the benefit of all the nice [fat] cream?"

It even made you feel guilty, robbing cream from babies. But now we know that we were doing our kids a favor —and ourselves an unfavor—by keeping the cream away from them.

There was also one other thing. You could tell the butterfat content of your milk by the proportion of cream that rose to the top of the bottle. Four percent butterfat gave a cream zone twice as big as two percent butterfat. That kept the dairymen honest, since they couldn't easily divert the cream you paid for to ice cream, butter, and other by-products, where they sold it to you all over again at a much higher price. But once the cream is all mixed with the milk, who knows what they're getting? Which brand of milk in your area has the most butterfat? You don't know. But if it weren't homogenized, you could tell from across the room. And anytime you wanted to mix the cream with the milk, all you had to do was shake the bottle. Good exercise. But there's more serious trouble with homogenized milk than that.

What kind of trouble?

Big big trouble. The process of homogenization consists of forcing the liquid through a very fine stainless-steel screen, with holes so small that the fat globules are broken down into tiny miniglobules which do not rise to the top of the milk.

It has been amply demonstrated that people who have heart attacks or serious arteriosclerosis have a marked decrease of a substance called *plasmalogen* in the cells of their bodies. Cow's milk contains a substance called *xanthine oxidase,* an enzyme. Now xanthine oxidase destroys plasmalogen and significantly increases the risk of severe heart attacks.

But then why doesn't everyone who drinks milk get a heart attack?

Because xanthine oxidase always hitches a ride on the large fat globules found in nonhomogenized milk. These globules are too big to be absorbed by the human intestine, and the xanthine oxidase in milk can't get into your body. But if you homogenize milk, you make the fat globules smaller, the xanthine oxidase slides into the body with ease, destroys the plasmalogen, and zap! The increased incidence of heart attacks in the United States exactly follows the increased use of homogenized milk. When you draw the two lines on a graph, they are almost parallel. In addition, people who drink *nonhomogenized* milk and still have heart attacks have a much lower death rate from their attacks. This doesn't mean that homogenized milk is the primary cause of heart attacks. However, it strongly suggests that it's another nail in your coffin. And remember, homogenizing milk only helps the giant milk companies. It doesn't do a thing for you—although it may do something *to* you.*

How do the dairy companies feel about that?

I asked a friend of mine in the dairy business what he thought about the hazards of homogenized milk. Do you know what he said? He said: "My God! It's taken us forty years to sell the idea of homogenized milk and you're going to undo it in two pages!" Do you think we'll be that lucky?

---

* Oster, K. A., Role of plasmalogen in heart disease, *Myocardiology: Recent Advanced Studies in Cardiac Structure and Metabolism.* Baltimore, University Park Press, 1973, Vol. I, pp. 803–815.

What kind of milk is safe to drink?

The only really safe milk is mother's milk until you're six months old. But if you like milk, the best milk is certified *nonpasteurized*, nonhomogenized milk from a nearby farm. "Certified" means that the cows are examined regularly and are free from disease; they get much better veterinary supervision than in the giant "milk-factory" commercial dairies, where they are given antibiotics in their feed instead of scrupulous sanitation. Certified milk has to be handled more carefully and kept germ-free until you buy it. Sterilized milk (also called "pasteurized") can be crawling with germs until they cook it and cover up all the sloppy handling. In European countries hundreds of millions of people drink certified unpasteurized milk every day—and they have fewer cases of milk-borne diseases than we do in the United States. Like homogenizing, pasteurizing makes bigger profits for dairies—not better milk for you.

If you can't find real natural milk—certified unpasteurized milk—then try for pasteurized unhomogenized. Tell the manager of your local dairy that's what you want, tell the supermarket manager, tell the owner of the corner market. You'll find it if you keep asking.

But grown-ups don't *need* milk.

What else can we drink?

Water, of course, but the only tap water that's really healthful is what you find high up in the mountains, where human sewage and chemical fertilizers and factory slop haven't gotten into your drinking supply. Probably the worst city in the United States for drinking water is New Orleans—through no fault of New Orleanians. Every city on the Mississippi dumps its sewage into the river—and that's what the folks down in New Orleans have to drink.

Get yourself a two-stage water filter: ceramic or cellulose plus activated charcoal.* Use that water for cooking and drinking. Drink tea and coffee but watch out for decaffeinated coffee, since the caffeine is extracted with powerful organic chemicals that may leave residues in your brain, liver, and muscles. Try fresh-squeezed fruit juices. And soda water—if you like it. But make your own soda water, since the commercial kind is full of a big slug of chemicals—yes, even plain old carbonated water. Buy a siphon bottle and a supply of carbon dioxide cartridges and you're in business for yourself.

What about fresh fruit and vegetables?

Superb, but remember to wash them well and/or soak them in a very mild detergent solution and then rinse thoroughly. The chemical hormones, pesticides, and fungicides that go on the fruit and vegetables shouldn't go into your body.

What about bread?

Eat bread made only with 100 percent stone-ground whole wheat flour, salt, yeast, and water. If you can't buy it that way, make it. If you think it's too much work, go in with your friends and take turns making it for each other. Only eat pies, cakes, cookies, spaghetti, macaroni, muffins, rolls, biscuits, and all the rest made with the same kind of flour. If you can't buy them, make them.

But what if I don't have time to make all that stuff?

If you don't have time now, you'll have time when you get out of the hospital—with diabetes, a heart attack, diverticulosis, or any of the dozen other diseases stupid eating brings on. I'm not kidding. These diseases don't

---

* Bottled water has two disadvantages: it is very expensive compared with the cost of filtering your own water, and you don't really know how good—or bad—it is.

happen by themselves—they are the direct result of eating harmful and denutrified food. Any well-trained and up-to-date doctor will confirm that for you.

You lock your doors against thieves, don't you? But a thief will only steal your property. Shouldn't you lock your body against bad foods that will steal your life?

What about desserts?

Desserts are fine but you have to use common sense. Take commercial ice cream, for instance. Where do you think they get the milk to make ice cream? In many dairy operations, it comes from what they call the "spoils"— outdated and stale milk returned from retail stores. Ice cream is so doped up with synthetic chemicals and artificial-imitation flavors you couldn't taste the rotten flavor of the sour milk anyway. And some companies have another nice trick. When the ice cream gets too old, the stores return it for credit and the dairy recycles it into more ice cream. That senile ice cream almost always ends up as one of America's favorites: chocolate. Why? Because chocolate covers up a spoiled flavor like nothing else. Yum-yum!

Don't eat cake from mixes, frosting from cans, puddings from powders, imitation whipped cream from aerosol cans, and all the assorted coagulated junk they sell you for "dessert." If you like cakes, make a cake using honey and whole wheat flour. You'll find it satisfies you, fills you fast, and won't make you fat. You can make pudding, pies, cookies, and dozens of other desserts that way without depriving yourself and without feeling guilty, and without harming your health—or the health of your children. If you go about it right, dessert can be as nutritious as the rest of your meal—and it can taste better than any of the chemistry-set combinations you see plugged on television.

But how do I learn to make all those new things?

Since you asked, I am in the process of writing a new cookbook that embodies all the principles of the ideal diet and the healthful ways of eating we have discussed in this book. If you're interested, drop me a postcard with your name and address—in care of Harold Matson Co., 22 East 40th Street, New York, N.Y. 10016—and I'll let you know when it's available—and the price.

What other foods are worth avoiding?

Don't eat any food that is pickled, smoked, salted, or otherwise preserved. Sausages, commercial hams, corned beef, bacon, smoked meats and smoked fish, and similar foods are little chemical laboratories that will keep sputtering within your body for years to come.

Various pickles and pickled vegetables are in the same category.

What about other kinds of meat?

Well, don't eat any meat that *you know* has been doped with diethylstilbestrol—DES.* Don't eat any meat that *you know* has been fed antibiotics. Don't eat chicken or poultry that *you know* has been fed antibiotics, hormones, or arsenic-containing feed. Don't eat any meat that *you know* has been frozen before it gets to you—*fresh* is the key word.

Fish is a sad story. There is more mercury in most fish than you should be eating. (Any amount of mercury is too much.) And besides, in the United States, over 90 percent of all fish sold is frozen at one time or another. It may be thawed when you buy it, but like the starlets on television, it probably isn't as young as it looks.

What about candy and chewing gum?

Chewing gum? It's fine if you like to chew what they sell you. Most chewing "gum" these days is either wax, plastic,

---

* You may have to import your meat from Canada, since Canada only allows its citizens to eat meat from the U.S. which is DES-free.

or rubber. It is saturated with refined sugar, and when you chew it you grind the rotten sugar into your teeth. Pretty soon you have—rotten teeth. But then at least you can't chew gum anymore.

Most commercial candy is fat, usually coconut oil, sweetened with massive amounts of refined sugar plus plenty of artificial flavoring and artificial coloring. If you like candy, make the good stuff yourself. The detailed recipes are in my forthcoming cookbook.

What about vitamin pills?

If you still think you need them, go back and read the chapters on vitamins and minerals again. I don't think you should take any pills or medicines of any kind—except the ones your doctor prescribes. And then you might ask him if they're absolutely necessary. When my patients ask me that question, I almost always find a way to cut down or eliminate the drugs they are taking.

What about health foods?

What about them? One of the greatest tragedies of modern life is that we have two kinds of places to buy food: *unhealth* food stores and *health* food stores. Ideally every food store should be a *health* food store. But every health food store isn't really a healthy place to buy food.

Some "health food stores" have their own section of cake mixes, instant protein drinks, canned foods, and all the rest of the junk items in a new dress. It's better than the supermarket but not as good as doing it the real way. The real way is fresh wholesome food honestly displayed and fairly priced. Some of the food co-ops in college towns come closest to honesty and fair-dealing in unprocessed and real food.

It seems to me that one of the best investments America could make would be to tear down half the hospitals and replace them with honest food stores.

And it took me twenty years as a practicing physician to realize that. . . .

What about food advertised on television?

Don't touch it. Remember that one minute of network advertising costs about $100,000—in prime time maybe as much as $200,000. Food processors can afford to advertise only food that has no real value. Think of the "food" that is advertised on TV and you'll know what I mean. Breakfast "cereal" costs less than the box it comes in; imitation-artificial, orange-flavored breakfast drink is cheaper to make than the fancy glass jar it comes in; those awful cake mixes are a few pennies' worth of refined flour, and on and on. You can't eat the TV ads—don't pay for them.

But how do I know that following the suggestions in this book will really help me?

Do you want a guarantee? Okay, here it is:
If you follow the suggestions in this book, you will eat better, you will save more money each month on food—for a family of four—than this book cost you, and you will give yourself and your family sound scientific protection against some of the most terrible diseases of modern civilization.
That's a promise.

Special Note to the Food Industry

You are going to hate this book and you are going to love it. You are going to hate it because you think it will hurt your profits—which is what big corporations care about the most. Let's be honest. You don't want me or anyone else to tell your 220 million customers that you have lied, deceived, and manipulated them unmercifully to make a fast buck. You don't want your customers to know how you influence Congress to pass the laws that will make big money for you at the expense of those who eat your products. You don't want the mommies and daddies of America to know how much it costs you to hype up *any* product —even this piece of paper—with 100 percent of the Recommended Adult Dietary Allowance of nine vitamins. (It costs you just about one fifth of a penny—according to your own trade journal, *Food Engineering*.)

You don't want anyone to know how bad and how dangerous the chemicals are that you heap into their food. You don't want them to know that so many of the chemical poisons you use are prohibited in other civilized countries. You don't want the people of your country to know that some of the foods they eat are of such rotten quality that they can't be sold to consumers in foreign countries. (Tell them about the pork and the chickens that we eat that other countries won't allow past their borders because of parasites, bad quality, and excessive water content.)

You hate this book so much that you're going to spend hundreds of thousands of dollars trying to discredit it. You're going to pay for sneering book reviews looking for little nitpicking errors. ("If Dr. Reuben is so smart, how come he doesn't know . . .") You're going to hire pay-for-play "experts" to "refute" this book. You're going to have your trade associations write threatening letters to try to intimidate anyone who has anything to do with the revelation of what you've been doing to us. Incidentally I'd be delighted to receive a copy of those threatening letters to add to my collection. Please send them to me, Dr. David Reuben, in care of Don Congdon of Harold Matson Co., 22 East 40th Street, New York, N.Y. 10016. I would appreciate it if you would write the words, "THREATENING LETTER" on the envelope so that it will go to the right place. All threatening letters will be promptly answered.

Now let me tell you why you're going to love this book. You will love it because you are sick of telling lies and twisting the truth. You're sick of selling food that can hurt people, especially little kids and pregnant mothers. You feel bad about snatching dollar bills from people for "fruit-flavored" drinks that are really only sugar and water and prevent poor people from eating real fruit. You feel bad because most of your customers for chemical imitation junk food are the poor people who believe all those little lies you tell them on television and in those subliminal full-page ads. You love this book because as individuals you are really decent people and you really do have a conscience, and this book tells the truth. And deep inside you know it is the truth.

So after you get over the first shock of facing reality, maybe you'll realize that being honest and fair and selling safe, nutritious food to your friends and your fellow Americans—and your own family—isn't such a bad idea after all. I hope you see it that way, because if you don't we are all in for some very bad times.

Special Note to the Food and Drug Administration

You're getting better but you have a long way to go. After exposing us to cyclamates, Red #2, diethylstilbestrol, nitrates and nitrites, saccharin, and a few hundred other deadly chemicals in our daily diet, you're getting the message.

You're starting to realize that your responsibility is *not* to the big food processors or the big chemical manufacturers or to any other big business. Your responsibility is to us—THE AMERICAN PEOPLE. We pay your salaries and free medical insurance and big retirement benefits. We provide those nice offices and fancy desks and the security of civil service. And speaking of service, your only reason to exist is to *serve us*. You are supposed to protect the helpless men, women, and children of this nation from all the crooks, chiselers, poisoners, and fast-buck artists of the world. Up to now, you've done a pretty rotten job—you know that better than anyone. It is inconceivable that less powerful and less technically sophisticated nations should be more advanced than us in protecting the food of their citizens. Shame on you!

I hope you will take the message in this book to heart. I hope you will correct your past mistakes. I hope you will remember that the responsibility for our health and safety

Everything You Always Wanted to Know About Nutrition

is in your hands. I hope you will remember that sooner or later you will have to account to the American people for the way you have done your job.

We depend on you. Don't let us down.

Bibliography

Ahart, H. E.: Assessing food intake of hospital patients. *J. Am. Dietet. A.*, 40:114, 1962.

Albrink, M. J.: Diet and cardiovascular disease. *J. Am. Dietet. A.*, 46:26, 1965.

Anderson, T. W., Reid, D. B. W., and Beaton, G. H.: Vitamin C and the common cold: A double-blind trial. *Canad. Med. Assn. J.*, 107:503, 1972.

Are all food calories equal? *Nutr. Rev.*, 22:177, 1964.

Arnaud, S., and Stickler, G.: Recent developments in vitamin D research. *Clin. Ped.*, 13:444, 1974.

Ayers, J. C., Kraft, A. A., Snyder, H. E., and Walker, H. W. (eds.): *Chemical and Biological Hazards in Food.* Ames, Iowa, Iowa State University Press, 1962.

Bagchi, K., Ray, R., and Datta, T.: The influence of dietary protein and methionine on serum cholesterol level. *Am. J. Clin. Nutr.*, 13:232, 1963.

Baker, E. M., et al.: Vitamin B_6 requirement for adult men. *Am. J. Clin. Nutr.*, 15:59, 1964.

Baker, E. M., Plough, I. C., and Allen, T. H.: Water requirement of men as related to the salt intake. *Am. J. Clin. Nutr.*, 12:394, 1963.

Berkowitz, D.: Metabolic changes associated with obesity before and after weight reduction. *J.A.M.A.*, 187:399, 1964.

Bieri, J.: Effect of excessive vitamins C and E on vitamin A status. *Am. J. Clin. Nutr.*, 26:382, 1973.

Bierring, W. L.: Preventive medicine: Its changing concepts—1859–1959. *J.A.M.A.*, 171:2190, 1959.

Brooke, M. M.: Epidemiology of amebiasis in the U.S. *J.A.M.A.*, 188:519, 1964.

Brown, E. B.: The absorption of iron. *Am. J. Clin. Nutr.*, 12:205, 1963.

Buja, L. M., and Roberts, W. C.: Iron storage disease. *Am. J. Med.*, 51:209, 1971.

Burke, B. S., et al.: Relationship between animal protein, total protein, and total caloric intakes in the diets of children one to eighteen years of age. *Am. J. Clin. Nutr.*, 9:136, 1961.

Burr, M.: Factors influencing the metabolic availability of ascorbic acid. *Clin. Pharmacol. & Therapeut.*, 18:238, 1975.

Burton, B. R. (ed.): *Heinz Handbook of Nutrition*, 2nd ed. New York, McGraw-Hill Book Company, 1965.

Butterworth, C.: Correcting malnutrition: Practical therapeutic approaches. *Mod. Med.*, Nov. 30, 1970, p. 97.

Callendar, S. T.: Iron absorption from food. *Geront. Clin.*, 13:44, 1971.

Campbell, J. A., and Morrison, A. B.: Some factors affecting the absorption of vitamins. *Am. J. Clin. Nutr.*, 12:162, 1963.

Cantarow, A., and Trumper, M.: *Clinical Biochemistry*, 6th ed. Philadelphia, W. B. Saunders Company, 1962.

Cardiovascular disease—the picture in the U.S. *J. Am. Dietet. A.*, 46:394, 1965.

Cereal Enrichment in Perspective, 1958. Prepared by The Committee on Cereals, Food and Nutrition Board, March 1958. National Academy of Sciences–National Research Council, Washington, D.C.

Chen, L. H., Liao, S., and Packet, L. V.: Interaction of dietary vitamin E and protein level or lipid source with cholesterol in the rat. *J. Nutr.*, 102:729, 1972.

Chien, L., Krumdieck, C., Scott, C., Jr., and Butterworth, C.: Harmful effect of megadoses of vitamins. *Am. J. Clin. Nutr.*, 28:51, 1975.

Chow, B. F., et al.: Diet and urinary output of water. *Am. J. Clin. Nutr.*, 12:333, 1963.

Clifton, J. A.: Intestinal absorption and malabsorption. *J. Am. Dietet. A.*, 39:449, 1961.

Clinical nutritional problems in the United States today. *Nutr. Rev.*, 23:1, 1965.

Cochrane, W. A.: Excessive administration of vitamins. *Canad. Med. Assn. J.*, 93:893, 1965.

Council report on dietary fat regulation. *Nutr. Rev.*, 21:36, 1963.

Coursin, D. B.: Undernutrition and brain function. *Borden's Review of Nutrition Research*, 26, No. 1, Jan.–Mar. 1965.

Cow's milk versus human milk protein in infant feeding. *Nutr. Rev.*, 20:67, 1962.

Crampton, E. W.: The philosophy of dietary standards (with particular reference to the adult requirements for energy and protein). *J. Canad. Dietet. A.*, 21:234, 1959.

Danielsson, H.: Influence of bile acids on digestion and absorption of lipids. *Am. J. Clin. Nutr.*, 12:214, 1963.

Darby, W.: Basic contributions to medicine by research in nutrition. *J.A.M.A.*, 180:816, 1962.

Darby, W.: The rational use of vitamins in medical practice. *Med. Clin. N.A.*, 48:1203, 1964.

Davidson, C. S., et al.: The nutrition of a group of apparently healthy aging persons. *Am. J. Clin. Nutr.*, 10:181, 1962.

DiCyan, E.: *Vitamin E and Aging.* New York, Pyramid Publications, 1972.

Diet, detoxification, and toxemia of pregnancy. *Nutr. Rev.*, 21:269, 1963.

Diet and growth in infancy, *Nutr. Rev.*, 21:327, 1963.

The diet of patients with arthritis. *Nutr. Rev.*, 21:203, 1963.

Digestion and absorption of disaccharides in man. *Nutr. Rev.*, 20:203, 1962.

Duncan, G. G. (ed.): *Diseases of Metabolism*, 5th ed. Philadelphia, W. B. Saunders Company, 1964.

Dunning, G. M.: Radioactivity in the diet. *J. Am. Dietet. A.*, 42:17, 1963.

Eadie, G. A., et al.: Type E botulism. *J.A.M.A.*, 187:496, 1964.

Ende, S. N.: Starvation studies with special reference to cholesterol. *Am. J. Clin. Nutr.*, 11:270, 1962.

Exton-Smith, A., and Scott, D. (eds.): *Vitamins in the Elderly* (Proceedings of a Symposium at the Royal College of Physicians, London). Bristol, John Wright & Sons, 1968.

FAO: Evaluation of the carcinogenic hazards of food additives. *FAO Nutrition Meetings Report*, Series 29; *WHO Tech. Rep.*, Series 220 (1961).

FAO: Procedures for the testing of intentional food additives to establish their safety for use. *FAO Nutrition Meetings Report*, Series 17: *WHO Tech Rep.*, Series 144 (1958).

FAO: Specifications for the identity and purity of food additives and their toxicological evaluation: Some emulsifiers and stabilizers and certain other substances. *FAO Nutrition Meetings Report*, Series 43; *WHO Tech. Rep.*, Series 373 (1967).

FAO: Specifications for the identity and purity of food additives and their toxicological evaluation: Some food colors, emulsifiers, stabilizers, anticaking agents, and certain other substances. *FAO Nutrition Meetings Report*, Series 46; *WHO Tech. Rep.*, Series 445 (1970).

FAO: Toxicology evaluation of some antimicrobials, antioxidants, emulsifiers, stabilizers, flour-treatment agents, acids and bases. *FAO Nutrition Meetings Report*, Series 40, A, B, C (1967).

FAO: Toxicology evaluation of some flavoring substances and non-nutritive sweetening agents. *FAO Nutrition Meetings Report*, Series 44A (1967).

FAO: Toxicological evaluation of some food colors, emulsifiers, stabilizers, anticaking agents and certain other substances. *FAO Nutrition Meetings Report*, Series 46A (1970).

Fat and cholesterol in the diet. *Nutr. Rev.*, 23:3, 1965.

Fluoridation in Great Britain. *Nutr. Rev.*, 21:99, 1963.

Folacin deficiency and alcoholism. *Nutr. Rev.*, 22:8, 1964.

Fomon, S. J., et al.: Calcium and phosphorous balance studies with normal full-term infants fed pooled human milk or various formulas. *Am. J. Clin. Nutr.*, 12:346, 1963.

Food additives. *Nutr. Rev.*, 19:227, 1961.

Freezer storage and vitamin stability in beef. *Nutr. Rev.*, 23:18, 1965.

Fry, P. C., et al.: Nutrient intakes of healthy older women. *J. Am. Dietet. A.*, 42:218, 1963.

Fullerton, D. T., Kollar, E. J., and Caldwell, A. B.: A clinical study of ulcerative colitis. *J.A.M.A.*, 181:463, 1962.

Furia, T. E. (ed.): *Handbook of Food Additives.* Cleveland, Chemical Rubber Company, 1968.

Gailani, S., Ohnuma, T., and Rosen, F.: Nutritional approaches to cancer therapy, in *Cancer Medicine*, Holland, E., and Frei, E., III (eds.). Philadelphia, Lea & Febiger, 1974.

Gastrointestinal protein loss in iron-deficiency anemia. *Nutr. Rev.*, 21:170, 1963.

Goodwin, R.: *Chemical Additives in Food.* London, Churchill, 1967.

Halac, E., Jr.: Studies of the relation between protein intake and resistance to protein deprivation. *Am. J. Clin. Nutr.*, 11:514, 1962.

Hardinge, M. G., Swarner, J. B., and Crooks, H.: Carbohydrates in foods. *J. Am. Dietet. A.*, 46:197, 1965.

Harrow, B., and Mazur, A.: *Textbook of Biochemistry*, 8th ed. Philadelphia, W. B. Saunders Company, 1962.

Hazards of overuse of vitamin D. A statement of the Food and Nutrition Board, National Academy of Sciences–National Research Council, Washington, D.C., Nov. 1974.

Hodges, R. E.: Experimental vitamin A deficiency in man. Western Hemisphere Nutrition Congress III, Miami Beach, 1971.

Hoffman, W. S., et al.: Pesticide storage in human fat tissue. *J.A.M.A.*, 188:819, 1964.

Holman, R. T.: How essential are fatty acids? *J.A.M.A.*, 178:930, 1961.

Hsu, J. M.: Effect of deficiencies of certain B vitamins and ascorbic acid on absorption of vitamin B_{12}. *Am. J. Clin. Nutr.*, 12:170, 1963.

Idiopathic ulcerative colitis and milk. *Nutr. Rev.*, 22:262, 1964.

Interrelationships between vitamins A and E. *Nutr. Rev.*, 23:82, 1965.

Iron storage in bone marrow. *Nutr. Rev.*, 21:329, 1963.

Johnson, B. C.: Dietary factors and vitamin K. *Nutr. Rev.*, 22:225, 1964.

Jolliffee, N. (ed.): *Clinical Nutrition,* 2nd ed. New York, Harper & Row, 1962.

King, B. G., and Showers, M. F.: *Human Anatomy and Physiology,* 5th ed. Philadelphia, W. B. Saunders Company, 1963.

Kinsell, L. W., et al.: Dietary considerations with regard to type of fat. *Am. J. Clin. Nutr.,* 15:198, 1964.

Kirsner, J. B.: Facts and fallacies of current medical therapy for uncomplicated duodenal ulcer. *J.A.M.A.,* 187:423, 1964.

Kramer, P., and Caso, E. K.: Is the rationale for gastrointestinal diet therapy sound? *J. Am. Dietet. A.,* 42:505, 1963.

Larrick, G. P.: The nutritive adequacy of our food supply. *J. Am. Dietet. A.,* 39:117, 1961.

Larson, R. H.: Effect of prenatal nutrition on oral structures. *J. Am. Dietet. A.,* 44:368, 1964.

Laureta, H. C., et al.: An appraisal of the management of peptic ulcer including comparative studies of the value of a polyunsaturated fat nutritional preparation in the management of gastric hypersecretion. *Am. J. Clin. Nutr.,* 15:211, 1964.

Mangay Chung, A. S., et al.: Folic acid, vitamin B_6, pantothenic acid and vitamin B_{12} in human dietaries. *Am. J. Clin. Nutr.,* 9:573, 1961.

Margolius, S.: *The Great American Food Hoax.* New York, Walker & Co., 1971.

Matoth, Y., et al.: Studies on folic acid in infancy. III. Folates in breast-fed infants and their mothers. *Am. J. Clin. Nutr.,* 16:356, 1965.

Maynard, L. A.: Effect of fertilizers on the nutritional value of foods. *J.A.M.A.,* 161:1478, 1956.

McMasters, V.: History of food composition tables of the world. *J. Am. Dietet. A.,* 43:442, 1963.

McOsker, D. E., et al.: The influence of partially hydrogenated dietary fats on serum cholesterol levels. *J.A.M.A.,* 180:380, 1962.

Mendel, G. A.: Iron metabolism and etiology of iron-storage diseases: An interpretive formulation. *J.A.M.A.,* 189:45, 1964.

The metabolic role of vitamin E. *Nutr. Rev.,* 23:90, 1965.

Miller, D., and Crane, R. K.: The digestion of carbohydrates in the small intestine. *Am. J. Clin. Nutr.,* 12:220, 1963.

Mitchell, H. S.: Protein limitation and human growth. *J. Am. Dietet. A.,* 44:165, 1964.

Moeller, H. C.: Conventional dietary treatment of peptic ulcer. *Am. J. Clin. Nutr.,* 15:194, 1964.

The most deadly poison. *J.A.M.A.,* 187:530, 1964.

Most, H.: Trichinellosia in the United States. *J.A.M.A.,* 193:871, 1965.

Moynahan, E. J., and Barnes, P. M.: Zinc deficiency and synthetic diet. *Lancet*, 1:676, 1973.

National Academy of Sciences: *Evaluating the Safety of Food Chemicals*, Publication No. 1859. Washington, D.C., 1970.

Nesheim, R.: Nutrient changes in food processing: A current review. *Fed. Proc.*, 33:2267, 1974.

Nitra, M.: Confusional states in relation to vitamin deficiencies in the elderly. *J. Am. Geriat. Soc.*, 19:536, 1971.

Nutritional cirrhosis of the liver. *Nutr. Rev.*, 21:175, 1963.

Nutrition Foundation: *Present Knowledge in Nutrition*, 3rd ed. New York, 1967.

Nutrition in preventive medicine. *Nutr. Rev.*, 7:1, 1950.

Olson, R. E.: The two-carbon chain in metabolism. *J.A.M.A.*, 183:471, 1963.

Pike, R. L.: Sodium intake during pregnancy. *J. Am. Dietet. A.*, 144:176, 1964.

Pincknev, E.: The potential toxicity of excessive polyunsaturates. *Am. Heart J.*, 85:723, 1973.

Protein and amino acid requirements. *Nutr. Rev.*, 20:235, 1962.

Rider, J. A., and Moeller, H. C.: Hypersensitivity factors in ulcerative colitis. *J.A.M.A.*, 183:545, 1963.

Roe, D. W.: Drug-induced vitamin deficiencies. *Drug Therapy*, 3:23, 1973.

Roehm, R. R., and Mayfield, H. L.: Effect of dietary fat on cholesterol. *Metabolism* 40:417, 1962.

Russell, R., Bover, J., Bagheri, S., and Hruban, Z.: Hepatic injury from chronic hypervitaminosis A resulting in portal hypertension and ascites. *N. Engl. J. Med.*, 291:435, 1974.

Salmonella control. *J.A.M.A.*, 189:691, 1964.

Sanchez, A., et al.: Nutritive value of selected proteins and protein combinations. I. The biological value of proteins singly and in meal patterns with varying fat composition. II. Biological value predictability. *Am. J. Clin. Nutr.*, 13:243; 13:250, 1963.

Sanders, H. J.: Food additives. *Chem. Eng. News,* October 10 and 17, 1966, p. 44.

Sandstead, H., Burk, E., Booth, G., and Darby W.: Current concepts on trace minerals. *Med. Clin. N.A.*, 54:1509, 1970.

Santini, R., et al.: The distribution of folic acid active compounds in individual foods. *Am. J. Clin. Nutr.*, 14:205, 1964.

Schaefer, A. E.: Nutritional deficiencies in developing countries. *J. Am. Dietet. A.*, 42:295, 1963.

Schroeder, H. A.: Losses of vitamins and trace minerals resulting from processing and preservation of foods. *Am. J. Clin. Nutr.*, 24:562, 1971.

Schultz, H. W.: Chemicals in foods. *J. Am. Dietet. A.*, 34:492, 1958.

Schwartz, W. S.: Management of common pulmonary diseases. *J.A.M.A.*, 181:134, 1962.

Scrimshaw, N. S.: Malnutrition and infection. *Borden's Review of Nutrition Research*, 26, No. 2, April–June 1965.

Seelig, M. S.: The requirement of magnesium by the normal adult. *Am. J. Clin. Nutr.*, 14:342, 1964.

Seymour, M.: Current practices, research and education in diet therapy. *Am. J. Clin. Nutr.*, 14:233, 1964.

Smith, A., and Kenyon, D. A.: Unifying concept of carcinogenesis and its therapeutic implications. *Oncology*, 27:459, 1973.

Smith, C. A.: Overuse of milk in the diets of infants and children. *J.A.M.A.*, 172:567, 1960.

Smith, E. H.: Problems in the safe and effective use of pesticides in agriculture. *Nutr. Rev.*, 22:193, 1964.

State, D.: Gastrointestinal hormones in the production of peptic ulcer. *J.A.M.A.*, 187:410, 1964.

Steiner, A., Howard, E. J., and Akgun, S.: Importance of dietary cholesterol in man. *J.A.M.A.*, 181:186, 1962.

Steinkamp, R. C., Choen, N. L., and Walsh, H.: Resurvey of an aging population—fourteen year follow-up. *J. Am. Dietet. A.*, 46:103, 1965.

Stitt, K. R.: Nutritive value of diets today and fifty years ago. *Nutr. Rev.*, 21:257, 1963.

Stone, D. B.: A rational approach to diet and diabetes. *J. Am. Dietet. A.*, 46:30, 1965.

Stowers, J. M.: Nutrition in diabetes. *Nutr. Abst. Rev.*, 33:1, 1963.

Symposium on human calcium requirements. *J.A.M.A.*, 185:588, 1963.

Tank, G.: Recent advances in dental caries. *J. Am. Dietet. A.*, 46:293, 1965.

Thompson, W. S.: World population and food supply. *J.A.M.A.*, 172:1647, 1960.

Tower, D. B.: Interrelationships of oxidative and nitrogen metabolism with cellular nutrition and function in the central nervous system. *Am. J. Clin. Nutr.*, 12:308, 1963.

Toxic reactions of vitamin A. *Nutr. Rev.*, 22:109, 1964.

Turner, D.: *Handbook of Diet Therapy*, 4th ed. Chicago, University of Chicago Press, 1965.

Udenfriend, S.: Factors in amino acid metabolism which can influence the central nervous system. *Am. J. Clin. Nutr.*, 12:287, 1963.

U.S. Dept. of Health, Education and Welfare: *Report of the Secretary's Commission on Pesticides and Their Relationship to Environmental Health* (the Mrak Report). Washington, D.C., 1969.

Vallee, B. L.: Clinical significance of trace elements. *Modern Medicine,* Feb. 18, 1963, p. 111.

Vought, R. L., and London, W. T.: Dietary sources of iodine. *Am. J. Clin. Nutr.,* 14:186, 1964.

Walker, A. P. R.: Anomalies in the prediction of nutritional disease. *Nutr. Rev.,* 19:257, 1961.

Walsh, H. E.: The changing nature of public health. *J. Am. Dietet. A.,* 46:93, 1965.

Watt, B. K., and Merrill. A. L.: *Composition of Food: Raw, Processed and Prepared.* U.S. Department of Agriculture, Agriculture Handbook Number 8, revised, 1963.

Weinstein, L., et al.: Diet as related to gastrointestinal function. *J.A.M.A.,* 176:935, 1961.

Weir, D. R., and Houser, H. B.: Problems in the evaluation of nutritional status in chronic illness. *Am. J. Clin. Nutr.,* 12:278, 1963.

WHO Report. *Calcium Requirement.* Technical Report No. 230, 1962.

Williams, H. H.: Differences between cow's and human milk. *J.A.M.A.,* 175:104, 1961.

Williams, R. J.: *Nutrition Against Disease.* New York, Pitman Publishing Co., 1971.

Wohl, M. G., and Goodhart, R. S. (eds): *Modern Nutrition in Health and Disease,* 3rd ed. Philadelphia, Lea & Febiger, 1964.

Wolf, G.: Some thoughts on the metabolic role of vitamin A. *Nutr. Rev.,* 20:161, 1962.

Woodruff, C. W.: Protein requirements of full-term infants. *J.A.M.A.,* 175:114, 1961.

Wurtman, R., and Fernstrom, J.: Effects of the diet on brain neurotransmitters. *Nutr. Rev.,* 32:193, 1974.

Wynder, E. L., and Day, E.: Some thoughts on the causation of chronic disease. *J.A.M.A.,* 175:997, 1961.

Yacowitz, H.: Urine excretion of minerals in obese humans on normal and high-protein low-calorie diets. Paper delivered at meeting of American Society of Experimental Biology, 1973.

Youmans, J. B.: The changing face of nutritional disease in America. *J.A.M.A.,* 189:672, 1964.

Ziporin, Z. Z., et al.: Vitamin content of foods exposed to ionizing radiation. *J. Nutr.,* 63:201, 1957.

Zukel, M. C.: Fat-controlled diets. *Am. J. Clin. Nutr.,* 16:270, 1965.

Index